Birth Control

An International Assessment

To the *few* who have made family planning programmes succeed, in the hope that their experience will come to help the *many* who are in need of services and information.

Birth Control

An International Assessment

Edited by Malcolm Potts & Pouru Bhiwandiwala
International Fertility Research Program

MTP PRESS LIMITED
International Medical Publishers

Published by
MTP Press Limited
Falcon House
Lancaster, England

Softcover reprint of the hardcover 1st edition 1979

British Library Cataloguing in Publication Data

Birth control.
1. Birth control
I. Potts, Malcolm II. Bhiwandiwala, Pouru
301.32'1 HQ766

ISBN 978-94-015-7287-3 ISBN 978-94-015-7285-9 (eBook)
DOI 10.1007/978-94-015-7285-9

Contents

List of Contributors vii

Preface ix
Fred O. Pinkham

1 Introduction 1
Malcolm Potts and Pouru Bhiwandiwala

SECTION ONE

Mother and Child

2 Family planning and health 17
Abdel Omran

3 Fertility and lactation 37
Jeroen van Ginneken

SECTION TWO

Successful Family Planning Programmes

4 Using the local community – Bali, Indonesia 55
Ida Bagus Astawa

5 Involving the community – Thailand 71
Mechai Viravaidya and Malcolm Potts

6 Involving the community – Howrah 93
Pouru Bhiwandiwala

7 **Taking family planning to the community – Bombay, India** 115
Datta Pai

8 **Social marketing – Sri Lanka and Bangladesh** 135
Terry Louis and Robert Ciszewski

9 **Self-sufficiency in family planning – Japan** 153
Chojiro Kunii

SECTION THREE

Barriers and Bottlenecks

10 **Female sterilization** 173
Pouru Bhiwandiwala

11 **Menstrual regulation** 187
Elton Kessel

12 **The abortion epidemic** 201
Hugo Corvalán

13 **Future developments in fertility control** 215
Roger Short

14 **Law and planned parenthood** 227
John Paxman and Rebecca Cook

15 **Resources for research** 255
Roy Greep

16 **Resources for programmes** 265
Nafis Sadik

SECTION FOUR

Conclusions

17 **Conclusions** 275
Malcolm Potts and Pouru Bhiwandiwala

Index 299

List of Contributors

Dr Ida Bagus Astawa,
Executive Chairman,
National Family Planning Coordinating Board,
Djl Melati – Denpasar,
Bali,
Indonesia

Dr Pouru Bhiwandiwala,
Assistant Medical Director,
International Fertility Research Program,
Research Triangle Park,
North Carolina 27709,
USA

Mr Robert L. Ciszewski,
Executive Director,
Population Services International,
110 East 59th Street,
Suite 1019,
New York,
New York 10022,
USA

Ms Rebecca J. Cook
Consultant,
Law and Planned Parenthood Programme,
International Planned Parenthood Federation,
18–20 Lower Regent Street,
London SW1Y 4PW,
England

Dr Hugo Corvalán,
UNFPA Regional Coordinator,
Carrera 11, No. 84–51,
Apartado Aéreo 091369,
Bogota,
Colombia

Dr Jeroen K. van Ginneken,
Department of Epidemiology,
Medical Research Centre,
PO Box 20752,
Nairobi,
Kenya

Dr Roy O. Greep,
Professor (Emeritus), Population Studies,
Harvard Medical School,
45 Shattuck Street,
Boston,
Massachusetts 02115,
USA

Dr Elton Kessel,
President,
International Fertility Research Program,
Research Triangle Park,
North Carolina 27709,
USA

Mr Chojiro Kunii,
Executive Director,
Japanese Organisation for International Cooperation in Family Planning,
Hoken Kaikan Bekkan,
1–1 Sadohara-cho,
Ichigaya, Shinjuku-ku,
Tokyo, Japan

Mr Terry Louis,
Director,
Population Services International,
56–12 Dhammarama Road,
Colombo 6,
Sri Lanka

LIST OF CONTRIBUTORS

Dr Abdel Omran,
Professor of Epidemiology,
School of Public Health,
University of North Carolina,
Chapel Hill,
North Carolina 27514,
USA

Dr Datta Pai,
Director,
Pearl Centre,
Senapati Bapat Marg,
Dadar, Bombay, 400028,
India

Mr John M. Paxman,
Consultant,
Law and Planned Parenthood
Programme,
International Planned Parenthood
Federation,
18–20 Lower Regent Street,
London SW1Y 4PW,
England

Dr Fred O. Pinkham,
National Chairman,
Population Crisis Committee,
1120 19th Street, NW
Washington DC 20036,
USA

Dr Malcolm Potts,
Executive Director,
International Fertility
Research Program,
Research Triangle Park,
North Carolina 27709,
USA

Dr Nafis Sadik,
Assistant Executive Director
and Chief,
Programme Division, UNFPA,
485 Lexington Avenue,
New York,
New York 10017,
USA

Dr Roger Short,
Director,
MRC Unit of Reproductive Biology,
Department of Obstetrics
and Gynaecology,
39 Chalmers Street,
Edinburgh EH3 9ER,
Scotland

Mr Mechai Viravaidya,
Director,
Community Based Family Planning
Services,
16 Sukhumvit Soi 14,
Bangkok,
Thailand

Preface

In less than three decades, the family planning movement has grown from a handful of dedicated individuals – some of whom went to jail for their open advocacy of birth control – to hundreds of national and international agencies, representing both governmental and private sectors. In recent years, international meetings such as those held at Bucharest and Tokyo have legitimized the concern over population growth voiced by early advocates such as William Draper and John D. Rockefeller III. These conclaves have confirmed the basic reproductive freedoms first championed by Margaret Sanger, Elise Ottesen-Jensen, Clarence Gamble, and other family planning pioneers.

Financial contributions from governments and private sources have increased steadily during the last decade, and many developing countries are now providing substantial resources of their own to implement and expand national family planning programmes. Truly, the rapid growth of the family planning movement worldwide has been one of the most impressive social phenomena of its kind in history.

The dramatic successes described in this volume show us that there are indeed a number of things that can be done to lower birth rates. But the populations of several countries will still inevitably double in less than 30 years. Today, despite fair to good economic progress in some regions; overcrowding, disease, environmental degradation, unemployment, insecurity, malnutrition and even famine continue to plague large segments of the developing world. Even with the best in development efforts, we will be running a catch-up race on all these fronts for decades to come.

On the population side, significant barriers to widespread family planning activities also still remain: the weakness of national and community leadership; the rudimentary character of those economic and administrative infrastructures through which information and services can be delivered; the persistence of conservative social and religious attitudes; and the absence of major new breakthroughs in contraceptive technology.

The greatest impediment to more rapid progress may well be our apparent inability to gauge our efforts to the sheer magnitude of the problem. If we continue to advance narrowly conceived linear solutions against the geometrically progressing population problem, we risk losing the battle. Both governmental and private sectors must jointly move beyond scattered demonstration projects to a massive franchisement of self-sustaining family planning programmes. Lowering birth rates in a neighbourhood through door-to-door delivery of contraceptives has proven to be an effective delivery method on a small scale. The larger task is to make a total range of supplies and services readily available to all citizens throughout a nation. Community-based distribution of contraceptive supplies must be matched with equally available community-based surgical services, and both must be made available on equitable terms to all citizens.

It is clear from the descriptions of successful programmes presented here by the editors, Doctors Malcolm Potts and Pouru Bhiwandiwala, that the spread of family planning services depends heavily upon local entrepreneurship and commitment. Most of the conditions for programme success which arise out of these examples are related in some way to the quality of local leadership. The cardinal conditions are:

* leadership of one or more indigenous entrepreneurs;
* direct community participation;
* demonstrated concern for the dignity and welfare of the individual;
* strong and consistent government support;
* private initiatives; and
* primary focus on making contraceptive information, supplies and services readily and humanely available to those who wish them.

Wide implementation of these principles would take us a long way towards a solution to the population problem, but this implies a special kind of commitment at every level of society. An inadequate effort at any level weakens the entire synergistic effect. *National governments* which are concerned with the impact of too-rapid population expansion on political stability and economic development must therefore espouse a strong national policy supporting responsible parenthood and back it with federal laws, policies, programmes, and budgets that encourage both public and private support throughout the national and local institutions. *Provincial governments,* which serve as coordinating and support units between national policies and local community activities, must share these population concerns and take responsibility and initiative in finding locally acceptable solutions. *City governments,* which are pressed by overcrowding, unemployment, unrest, and strained public services must recognize the need to use existing and suitable urban infrastructures for the provision of family planning information and services. If ready-made mechanisms for delivery of family planning services do not exist, new specialized systems must be created.

The first concerns of *villages* are usually clean water supply, food production, housing, and provision of other fundamental necessities for rural living. Their role in support of family planning is central, for they are the point of direct political and economic contact for the majority of citizens in developing countries. The village must, therefore, provide critical frontline structures and channels through which family planning supplies and services can be provided. *Families,* quite naturally, are most interested in the health and security of the familial group. As societies 'modernize', strong cultural codes give way to new ideas which entail greater self-reliance and responsibility. Therefore, full attention should be given to the changing family relationship to the community and to the personal welfare, dignity and right to fulfilment of each person in the family. At each level, enlightened self-interest must underpin the continuum of direct and purposeful actions designed to bring birth rates into line with the desires and potentials for a better life. Central to the whole movement must be an understanding and genuine regard for each person. It is the welfare of the *individual,* after all, that is the ultimate concern. Where this continuum of commitment and concern exists – from the national cabinet down to the village council and family circle – adequate resources become available, and all of the presumed barriers to widespread contraceptive use melt away.

While the magnitude of the task remains mind-boggling, we are not without good and clear solutions. Signs of progress, as seen in the excellent programmes described herein, are surfacing in increasing numbers. Hopefully, we are now finding ways to create self-regenerating programmes which will spawn new efforts which, in turn, will drive other programmes forward, thus producing the momentum required to overcome population growth.

If the ravages of overpopulation are overcome, it will be because talented local citizens everywhere heeded the call of the family planning pioneers, followed their example, and built upon their contributions. While each locale must develop its own precise formula from its own unique setting, the illustrative programmes and commentaries in this book should provide encouragement for intensified action by national and local leaders committed to defusing the population bomb.

Fred O. Pinkham
National Chairman
Population Crisis Committee

1

Introduction

Malcolm Potts
and
Pouru Bhiwandiwala

POPULATION PROBLEMS AND PROGRAMMES 1
BUCHAREST AND TOKYO 3
CURRENT SITUATION 7
SUCCESSFUL AND UNSUCCESSFUL PROGRAMMES 8
THE PRIVATE SECTOR 11
ACTION NOW! 12

POPULATION PROBLEMS AND PROGRAMMES

The facts of the population explosion are well known. The changes in death rates which have occurred since the end of the Second World War have led to a doubling of population in many developing countries. Much of the real progress that has been made in agricultural production and economic development has been eroded by increasing numbers of people requiring food and employment. A second doubling of the population is forecast in some countries by the year 2000 AD, if present fertility rates remain unchanged. In 1976, the world population exceeded the four billion mark and every year there is an additional increase of 70 million people.

Most of the world's population is poor and likely to remain so. At present, the majority of the world's people still live in rural areas, but by 2000 AD the majority will live in towns and 40% in large cities (Figure 1). However, they are likely to remain poor with most of the additional population living in slums and shanty towns.

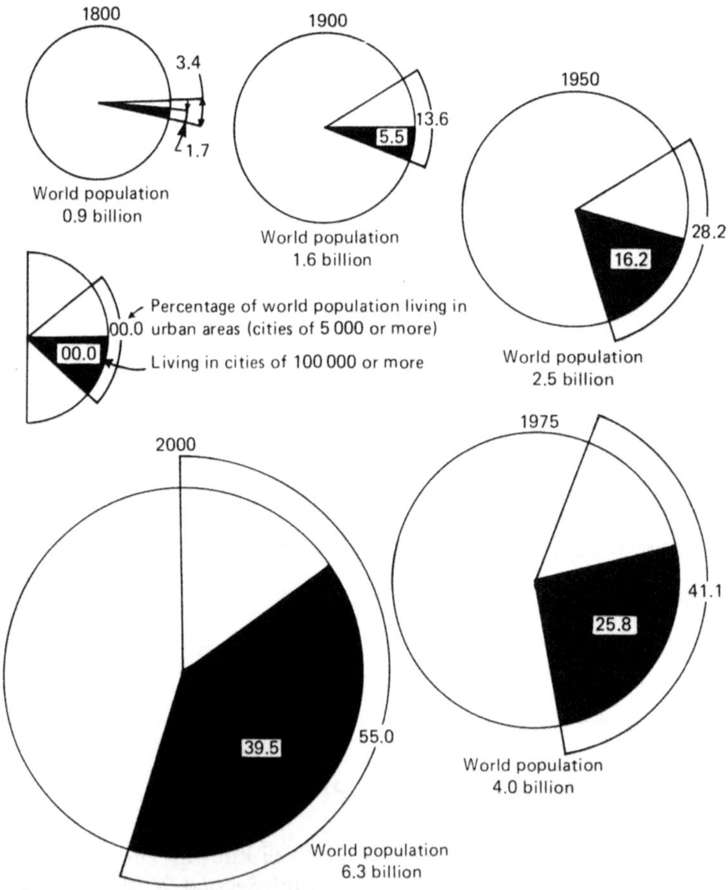

Figure 1 Changing percentage of world population living in urban and rural areas

In many countries half the population or more is below the age of marriage: the children born in the population explosion of the 1950s and 1960s will soon become parents themselves. In some countries there are as many first-born babies as there are deaths to adults and even if a two-child family were to prevail immediately, human numbers would continue to grow. No amount of family planning can alter the broad base of the population pyramid that now exists in the developed world and although birth *rates* may be falling, the absolute *increment* to the population is either steady or continuing to rise. The purpose of this volume is to review the biological, technical, managerial and funding problems that face family planning and to ask what are the main bottlenecks which exist at the present time.

The core of the book consists of accounts of successful family planning programmes written by people who initiated and conducted them during key phases of development. Programmes have been selected from governmental and non-governmental agencies, from developed and developing countries and include the surgical means of fertility control as well as the distribution of the reversible means of contraception. Attention is focused mainly on programmes which have been successful in extending meaningful family planning choices to poor communities. An attempt is made to ask what are the characteristics leading to success in these situations so as to be able to face the challenge of replicating such programmes at significant national levels.

Some of the projects discussed have had a dramatic impact on local population growth and the theme that emerges is that perhaps we know more about how to run successful family planning programmes than is sometimes realized. Often people are ahead of the decision makers, administrators and physicians involved in services and appear ready and sometimes even eager to adopt effective means of fertility regulation. Since 1974 the World Fertility Survey has conducted sample surveys in many developing countries which demonstrate current attitudes towards childbearing and the use of contraceptive practices and enable recent fertility changes to be analysed. As more couples use contraceptives so more want fewer children (Table 1).

As in any human activity, choices are usually based on a mixture of facts and opinions. Family planning has often proved a controversial subject and therefore has attracted individualists with strong opinions. Our analysis and the choice and content of some of the later contributions to this volume are not necessarily universally accepted, but it is hoped that they will prompt discussion in key areas concerning one of the most critical problems facing mankind today.

BUCHAREST AND TOKYO

The biology of human reproduction and the sociology of control of human fertility were some of the last areas to come under objective scientific surveillance. The individuals who first prompted the concept of family planning

TABLE 1 Desired and achieved family size, contraceptive use and fertility decline in six developing countries

	South Korea	*Thailand*	*Pakistan*	*Dominican Republic*	*Nepal*	*Malaysia*
Total fertility rate* 1965	4.6	6.6	7.5	7.4	—	5.6
1974	3.6	4.9	6.3	4.8	6.8	4.7
Percentage decline TFR 1965–74	21	25	16	37	—	16
Desired family size	3.2	3.7	4.3	4.8	3.9	4.4
Percentage wanting no more children†	72	57	49	45	30	43
Percentage using a contraceptive method	46	37	6	38	3	37
Principal methods used:						
Pills and injectables	10	17	1	—	—	16
Sterilization (male and female)	6	9	1	—	—	7
IUD	9	7	1	—	—	1
Percentage of women who have never heard of a contraceptive	3.0	4.0	25.0	2.5	77.6	8.1

* Total fertility rate (TFR): the number of children an average woman is likely to have in her lifetime at current fertility rates.

† Percentage based on currently married women aged 15–44.

Modified from Brackett, Ravenholt and Chao, 1978

or drew attention to the problems that might arise from expanding populations often found they had espoused an unpopular cause. It took several decades for political leaders to feel sufficiently confident to be able to establish policies in family planning and population. For a long interval the only funds available were those that came from private sources. Problems still remain and, although the majority of developing countries now have population and family planning policies, in some they are framed in consciously vague terms and programmes can still shy away from key issues for fear of arousing disapproval.

Much of the early effort in family planning, particularly in the developing world, was fuelled by an awareness and fear of the population explosion. However, there was always a significant group of people whose judgement was more sanguine. On occasions, frank warfare broke out between enthusiasts promoting family planning and more conservative elements within society. As family planning has matured, its vision has broadened and these debates, while still present and significant, have become less intense.

Shadows of former debates, however, were still present at the time of the Bucharest World Population Conference in 1974. The Conference itself concentrated on awareness and education, not on the design of services. In the words of Rafael Salas, Executive Director, United Nations Fund for Population Activities (UNFPA), there were 'a series of acrimonious exchanges on the proper weight to be assigned to the influence of rapid population growth on economic change and how it should be dealt with'. Yet the conference went on to develop a unanimous concern with family planning as a basic human right:

> 'All couples and individuals have the basic right to decide freely and responsibly the number and spacing of their children and to have the information, education and means to do so; the responsibility of couples and individuals in the exercise of this right takes into account the needs of their living and future children and their responsibilities towards the community.'

Like many human rights which are easy to state, the right to determine family size is a difficult one to implement. Millions of couples are beyond the reach of modern family planning services. The International Planned Parenthood Federation (IPPF) estimated, on the basis of an unmet needs study in 1976, that among over 550 million women at risk for pregnancy in the world, more than 260 million were not protected by the use of any method of family planning. The greatest numbers of couples in need of family planning were in relatively few countries (India, Indonesia, Brazil, Nigeria, Bangladesh, Pakistan and Mexico). The main part of this book looks at programmes which could act as models to fill these vast unmet needs.

Three years after Bucharest, a less publicized but equally interesting non-governmental initiative took place in Tokyo. Representatives of many disciplines, including economics, urban and rural development, health, child welfare, social and humanitarian agencies came together with a group of technically informed workers in family planning to review the current status of programmes and their impact. The Symposium made a number of action recommendations:

* to make the fullest range of family planning services available in rural areas and marginal districts of cities;
* to expand the social and economic roles of women and to improve their status in other fields;

* to educate adolescents and young adults about their reproductive behaviour and to underscore the impact premature parenthood would have on themselves, their families and their communities;
* to integrate family planning services with developmental activities, where this will benefit the community and its members;
* to place the responsibility and authority for programme design, implementation and funding as close as possible to the people affected.

A small specialized meeting organized by the International Fertility Research Program (IFRP) preceded the Tokyo Symposium and was linked to it. The publication that came out of that meeting, *Taking Family Planning to the World's Poor,* aroused considerable interest and, to some extent, this volume builds on these earlier meetings, expanding and documenting certain arguments in greater detail. Several of the contributors to this volume participated in the IFRP meeting which was held in Colombo (1977).

Conference quotations

"Family planning always begins in a controversial environment."

"Really, the international agencies are spending millions of dollars not so much to help people plan their families as to make the controversial aspects of the work politically respectable."

"Family planning always begins with the least relevant programmes and devices and then gradually develops."

"The law is always ten years behind you."

"We offer people not what they want but what we are able to give them politically."

"There are workshops, taskforces, this, that, and the other, but in the big field programmes things just aren't there."

"It is oppression, suppression and compression all the way – our conditions are so difficult I could sit down and weep."

– Colombo, 1977 –

CURRENT SITUATION

The benefits to social and economic development of reducing current rates of population growth are widely recognized and the whole world now accepts, without reservation, the important health consequences for the individual mother and her family of the optimum timing of births. These health benefits are many and varied as is apparent in Chapter 2.

In general terms, family planning often began with the least effective methods and programmes for the very reason that these were also the least challenging politically. The common evolution of family planning services has been to pass through a stage where private physicians helped the urban middle classes, on to one where voluntary, non-governmental family planning associations attempted to extend services to the poor, before finally reaching the stage of governmental policies and government financed or subsidized services. In the case of the developing world, the funding for the second stage often came partly from developed nations, particularly through the IPPF, which although now supported almost entirely by governments, was launched by private donations, largely from the USA and in great measure due to the efforts of one man – the late William Draper.

Physicians became involved in family planning at an early stage in its history for a number of reasons. Their work gave them a particularly vivid insight into the burdens of excess fertility and their skills were technically necessary for certain tasks. But they also had another role – they made it possible to package family planning services in a politically acceptable form. Margaret Sanger was well aware of the respectability which doctors offered her fledgling movement in the USA, although at that time vaginal barrier methods were largely offered, which as Marie Stopes showed in Britain, could be adequately taught by nurse practitioners.

One consequence of the controversy during the past decade which so often ranged around family planning is that those who first launched services saw them as a more novel undertaking than they have actually proved to be. It is now apparent that nearly every human community regulates its fertility. Even in developing countries with high birthrates, the achieved family size is often 6, 7 or 8 children and not the 10, 11 or 12 which is the *average* for unregulated human fertility.

In traditional societies and in pre-industrial Europe, human fertility has been limited in response to social and economic pressures by means of delayed marriage, traditional family planning techniques (such as *coitus interruptus*), induced abortion and breast feeding. Lactation is nature's contraceptive which adjusts reproduction to an optimum output. In mammals which breed throughout all seasons, lactation determines the interval between two conceptions.

In traditional societies, women breast feed for one or two years and for much of this time ovulation is suppressed. A considerable part of the practice of contraception in the modern world is no more than replacing the part previously played by breast feeding. Any unnecessary acceleration of the trend towards bottle feeding which accompanies urbanization and modern living, will aggravate existing problems of fertility control. The relationship between fertility and lactation is discussed in Chapter 3.

Other areas have, until recently, also been largely left outside the orbit of those interested in family planning. Statute law often embodies the rules which society evolved to regulate human sexual and reproductive behaviour in another age with different needs. Today, a number of countries are reviewing laws concerning the age at marriage, inheritance, access to contraception and the regulation of voluntary sterilization and induced abortion. An increasingly significant body of opinion is emphasizing the close relationship between the status of women within a society and the desire and opportunity to use new choices in fertility regulation. These are large and complicated themes that cannot be worked out in detail in a single volume but the relationship between law and population has been chosen for further analysis (Chapter 14). Some of the technical aspects of creating family planning programmes, such as the experience of social marketing in Bangladesh by Population Services International (Chapter 8) and of contraceptive distribution in Calcutta (Chapter 5), suggest practical ways of extending help to individuals in communities where women are unlikely to achieve social equality in the next one or two generations.

SUCCESSFUL AND UNSUCCESSFUL PROGRAMMES

In limited areas of the developing world, fertility is beginning to decline moderately rapidly (Table 1). Outside the Peoples' Republic of China, the changes that have occurred are not necessarily on a large scale and have certainly not made a numerically significant contribution to the world's problems. At the same time, they are not trivial. The successful programmes analysed in this volume involve moderately comprehensive services to 2.3 million people in Bali, Indonesia, village-based family planning services in Thailand which are currently being extended to cover fifteen million people, and social marketing of the reversible methods of contraception to the whole of Sri Lanka (population 14 million) and Bangladesh (population 84 million).

Other examples which could have been quoted include the remarkable changes which have occurred in Chiang Mai and Chiang Rai in the north of Thailand. Here a programme which began around the injectable contraceptive, Depo-Provera, but now includes the distribution of Pills and the option of sterilization, has been associated with a decline in mean family size from over 6 to 2.8 and a fall in the birth rate from 32 to 18/1000 in 13 years. In Colombia, Latin America, a similar change has taken place. Community-based village family planning programmes of the type described in Thailand (Chapter 5) were pioneered in Colombia and a large population is now served in that country. Big programmes have been successfully implemented in Brazil. The government programme which has been so successful in Bali is also extending throughout Indonesia. Unfortunately, for every successful programme several others have failed. In one relatively small Asian country US $8 million were injected into the family planning programme between 1974 and 1977, yet the number of new acceptors of family planning actually *declined* by half.

At a national level, many observers believe that the Peoples' Republic of China has made more progress in family planning than any other large nation in the developing world. In so vast and diverse a country a uniform response

TABLE 2 Chang Ching (Evergreen) Peoples' Commune, Soochow, China*

Population (1976)	19 502
Births	329
Birth rate	16.9/1000
Deaths	109
Natural increase	1.1%
Number of married women of reproductive age	2710
Number of unmarried women of reproductive age	720
Female sterilizations	1133
Male sterilizations	487
IUDs	493
Oral contraceptive users	251
Pregnant and nursing women	346
Percentage of eligible women using contraceptives	87%

* Jaffe 1977

to a family planning programme is unlikely. But there is compelling evidence that in many agricultural communes (Table 2) and in most urban areas birth rates have fallen significantly.

The political and cultural behaviour of contemporary China is so very different from Asia, Africa and Latin America that it is easy to argue that it is a special case. However, there are some interesting common factors with other successful programmes in developing countries. China makes available the full range of fertility regulation methods. In this it is unique in going further than any other country, except for Singapore. Pills and condoms are accessible to all married couples. Sterilization is available electively and abortion is easy to obtain and undoubtedly widely used, although not always listed prominently by the Chinese themselves. A genuine and apparently successful effort has been made to raise the age of marriage. Perhaps the unusual thing about China is that, whereas in other countries public advertisement and family planning motivation have been extensively employed, in China (which is in many ways a very puritan society), social pressures from within small communes have been used to influence individuals. But even here it is easy to overlook common factors with other countries of different political persuasions. The type of social pressure which appears to be exerted upon a married couple in China to have a prescribed number of children, in certain ways may be comparable to that which is exerted on an unmarried girl in other countries not to have children at all. It is a social pressure not necessarily backed up by physical or legal compulsion, but one which is strongly felt and carries a real emotional and status penalty for anyone who breaks the established conventions.

Those who have contributed programme descriptions to this volume come from many backgrounds but, as will become apparent, there are often more similarities than differences between successful programmes. Although family planning is a topic which attracts a great many conferences and working groups, those involved in implementing the programmes at the field level are not asked their experience and opinions as often as might be useful. Contrary to the popular assumption that the main barrier to taking family planning services to the world's poor lies in their lack of response, the experience of field managers is often that the major bottlenecks in family planning are political and administrative rather than reluctance on the part of the potential consumer to use contraceptives.

Inside a country, strong political backing is essential for successful family planning programmes, as the example of Indonesia shows in such a positive way. The ideal desired by programme managers is to have a national policy unanimously endorsed by all parties, but kept free of political considerations and passed down through all levels of the administration, religious leadership and community. Indifference or opposition within political leadership particularly affects the range of methods and type of personnel to be used. Generally, the more conservative the political climate, the less likely it is that there will be free access to the surgical methods of family planning and the more likely it is that managers will be compelled to utilize more highly qualified personnel than the techniques demand. When programmes lack political backing, their promotion and advertising which are essential for success are difficult. When opposition is extreme, the service may even be forced to maintain a low profile to avoid provoking a backlash.

The second bottleneck which programme managers identify, commonly concerns the way available resources are transmitted to field programmes. The record suggests that the freedom to follow businesslike management principles, to adjust programmes and therefore budgets to meet new demands and new opportunities and the degree of security and confidence which field personnel feel in the donor are all essential elements to success. It is recognized that many potential donors, particularly governmental and intergovernmental agencies, have to work within certain restraints. Therefore, attention has to be given to constructive ways of bridging the potential gap between the political and bureaucratic constraints within which many donors have to work and the need for freedom and flexibility which is essential to successful family planning programmes, must be recognized.

Behind every successful programme is an individual. Family planning is a topic where a few individuals *can* change a nation. Mr Chojiro Kunii's account of self-sufficient family planning services (Chapter 9) flows naturally from his own personal involvement in a situation where two out of three Japanese never used a contraceptive in 1950 to a state where six out of seven practise contraception today. Datta Pai offered sterilization to the poor with a directness that offended the rich when he first began. Mechai Virvaidya, with his incessant emphasis on contraceptives, has been so successful in getting his message across that his name 'Mechai' has become the popular name for a condom. But such changes are not achieved without controversy and sometimes frank unpopularity for those involved. Often, the courageous band of individuals who bring family planning out of the bedroom and into the market place and the public debating chamber work within non-governmental organizations.

THE PRIVATE SECTOR

One of the themes which emerged at the Tokyo Symposium and is emphasized in a number of places in this volume, concerns the role of non-governmental organizations and funds in family planning. Private initiatives have almost invariably preceded governmental involvement in family planning and have often charted the way that governments were to follow some years later. It is sometimes forgotten that in most developed countries birth rates fell in the absence of any structured government programme. This is not to say that a more humane and acceptable transition from high to low fertility would have been achieved had the community extended humane resources to citizens attempting to control their fertility. Undoubtedly, in western countries, illegal abortion played a significant factor in the decline of fertility which has taken place over the last hundred years. The rational involvement of government facilities now found in Scandinavia, Britain or Yugoslavia would have benefited the community one or two generations earlier. Nevertheless, it is interesting to look at the record of community self-help and do-it-yourself activities in family planning. In Japan, even at the present time, the government contributes no more than a few cents per capita to family planning activities. The record of the Japanese Family Planning Association and the current structure of fertility regulation services in Japan is an interesting one and for this reason Japan is the only developed country whose family planning services are reviewed in this volume (Chapter 9).

Strategies need to be developed to ensure that governmental and private agencies use their potential strengths to the best effect. In poor countries where government resources are overstretched and must cover a great many demanding human needs, it is also common sense to look towards some degree of self-sufficiency in family planning services. In this volume the role of social marketing, which returns some but not all the income necessary to run effective distribution services for the reversible methods, is highlighted (Chapter 8). The pioneer experience of not-for-profit, private sector, effectively managed surgical clinics in India also provides an example which is worth analysing in detail (Chapter 7). This type of clinic which depends on the entrepreneur manager and which coordinates and utilizes private doctors as cost-effectively as possible has its parallels in a number of other countries such as Thailand, Taiwan, the Philippines, Nigeria and Mexico. It is a concept which has been particularly promoted by International Pregnancy Advisory Services (IPAS).

ACTION NOW!

The 1977 Tokyo Symposium called for 'Action now towards more responsible parenthood worldwide'. What are the key areas for action? The growth in the world's population with the pressures it puts on development, employment, urbanization and ultimately on the carrying capacity of the fragile biosphere of the planet is not going to cease suddenly. The broad base to the population pyramid that now exists in the developing world has been noted: for every woman who reaches the menopause there are often two brides entering the fertile age group. Yet immediate changes in births, even if modest in amount, will exert great long term leverage. The problem facing many countries is not whether their population will double, but whether it will triple or more.

A scientific breakthrough which will suddenly produce 'the perfect contraceptive' is unlikely. The development, testing and introduction of new methods of fertility control, as is pointed out in Chapter 13, is necessarily slow. No one method is ever likely to be pre-eminently successful. This is not to say that contraceptive research is an unimportant area, but all the evidence is that it is becoming seriously underfunded (Chapter 15). Nor should we overlook the opportunity of tailoring existing methods of contraception more fully to differing cultural needs.

However, the prime emphasis of this volume is on immediate achievable decisions that will hasten the goal of extending family planning choices to all people and especially to the world's poor. It is our sincere hope that by trying to understand successful programmes, by listening to what the managers of programmes have to say and, above all, by attempting to respond to the needs and perceptions of people who are trying to control births, that we will help stimulate the policy and management decisions necessary to extend help to those currently without choice in that most basic of human functions – reproduction.

Bibliography

Abel Smith, B. (1974). *People without Choice.* (London: IPPF)

Bailey, J. and Correa, J. (1975). Evaluation of the Profamilia rural family planning programme. *Studies in Family Planning,* **6,** 148

Echeverry, G. (1975). Development of the Profamilia rural family planning program in Colombia. *Studies in Family Planning,* **6,** 142

Henderson, J. (1978). IPPF survey of unmet needs in family planning (1971–76). *People,* **5,** 25

Jaffe, F. S. and Oakley, D. (1978). Observations on birth planning in China 1977. *Family Planning Perspectives,* **10,** 101

Potts, M., Kessel, E. and Bhiwandiwala, P. (1977). *Taking Family Planning to the World's Poor.* (North Carolina : IFRP)

Salas, R. M. (1976). *People – An International Choice.* (Oxford: Pergamon Press)

SECTION ONE

Mother and Child

The ill effects of too rapid population growth on economic and social development are well recognized. The costs of reproduction for the individual mother's health have been known for a long time, but their full analysis is more recent. Were it necessary, they would more than justify family planning programmes of themselves.

The major biological variables affecting maternal and child health are straightforward: pregnancy interval, maternal age, and number of previous pregnancies. Important socio-economic variables include income and legitimacy. The impact of these factors is widespread and complex, such as differences in the chance of death or complication at delivery for both mother and baby and variations in long term outcome, even including differences in intellectual performance in the offspring. There is a limited span in the fertile life of a woman, and a balance in pregnancy number and spacing that defines when reproduction should take place for optimum safety and maximum probability of health in the next generation.

Breast feeding is nature's contraceptive and, in traditional societies, establishes an appropriate interval between conceptions. A proportion of the contraceptive practice of a modern country merely substitutes for the protection once given by lactation. In the developing world, there is a danger that bottle feeding will spread more rapidly than family planning services, compounding the serious problems of fertility regulation that already exist.

2

Family planning and health

Abdel Omran

INTRODUCTION	18
The fertility profile of the world	18
The health rationale for family planning	20
FAMILY PLANNING AND CHILD HEALTH	21
Parity and birth order effect	21
Effect of birth interval	22
Timing of pregnancy	22
Health risks to survivors	23
Effect on intellectual development	23
FAMILY PLANNING AND MATERNAL HEALTH	24
Increased maternal mortality	24
Increased obstetric risks	25
Increased non-obstetric conditions	25
FAMILY PLANNING AND TEENAGE PREGNANCY	26
The problem of rising teenage pregnancy	27
Health hazards of teenage pregnancy	27
FAMILY PLANNING METHODS AND HEALTH	27
LACTATION AND HEALTH	28
FAMILY PLANNING AND INFERTILITY	29
FAMILY PLANNING AND HEALTH DELIVERY SYSTEMS	29
IMPACT OF CHILD LOSS ON FERTILITY LEVEL	31

THE ACCEPTABILITY OF THE HEALTH RATIONALE FOR FAMILY PLANNING 32

CONCLUSIONS 32

INTRODUCTION

The fertility profile of the world

High fertility accompanied by declining mortality is at the root of the world's population problem. Ironically, the countries with ample resources and developed technology are those in control of their fertility. Countries with less developed technology are still unable to control their fertility or decrease their

Table 1 Demographic indicators of the world and its regions

Region	*Crude birth rate (per 1000 population) 1970–75*	*Total fertility rate (per 1000 women aged 15–49) 1970–75*	*Population (in 1000s) mid-1975*	*Rate of population growth (%) 1970–75*	*Years to double population*
World	31.5	4357	3 967 864	1.89	37
LDC	37.5	5267	2 836 180	2.31	30
MDC	17.2	2327	1 131 684	0.86	80
Africa	46.3	6309	401 314	2.64	26
Latin America	36.9	5265	324 092	2.71	26
East Asia	26.2	3594	1 006 380	1.65	42
South Asia	41.9	5981	1 249 793	2.63	27
Europe	16.1	2295	473 098	0.60	115
North America	16.5	2205	236 841	0.90	77
Oceania	24.8	3412	21 308	1.95	35
USSR	17.8	2417	255 038	0.99	70

Source: Selected World Demographic Indicators for the UN Secretariat, 1970–75

high rate of population growth. About three-quarters of the world population live in these less developed regions where the average birth rate is 37.5 per 1000 population compared to only 17.2 in the more developed regions. A woman in the third world would net, on the average, 5–6 children during her lifespan compared to only two children per woman in the more developed regions. In many countries in Africa, Asia and Latin and Middle America (Table 1), the birth rate exceeded 45 per 1000, and a woman would net 6–8 children.

The population of such a high fertility would require a special detailed sociological analysis. Briefly, there are prominent reasons for continuing high fertility in the developing countries.

(a) For centuries, high fertility was a necessity especially in the less developed regions in response to extremely high mortality. In face of devastating epidemics, wars and famines, the birth rate had to be kept high to assure family, tribal or national survival.

(b) High mortality in the Third World usually takes its greatest toll among children and young adults. Children and young adults are the most valued segments of the population in these regions since they are the sources for social, economic, and emotional security for their parents and for the community at large. Hence, fertility was kept high to insure that an enough number of children, especially sons will survive. This is perhaps a necessity in agrarian societies where the predominant character of labour is manual, and where a family's wealth is dependent upon the number of hands that can be put to work.

(c) Children are also a source of security for the mother, in particular against divorce or sharing her husband with another wife.

(d) In certain societies, particularly India, local cultural and religious beliefs require that at least one son should survive his parents in order to perform specific religious rituals after their death. Hence the predominant preference for sons in India.

(e) Marriage is a universal institution in the Third World, and young age at marriage especially for girls is the rule even until today in many societies. This is more prominent in Muslim societies, where premarital relations are not sanctioned and where the family's honour would be at stake if a girl were not married soon after puberty. This is also common in other countries like India, where marriages are usually arranged especially for girls, and where marriages are actually contracted for even before a girl reaches puberty. In absence of contraception, young age at marriage means longer period of exposure to pregnancy.

(f) This is compounded further by the social pressure, especially from mothers-in-law, on a bride to have a child as soon after marriage as possible as a proof of her fecundity, and of her husband's virility as well.

For these and other reasons, family planning needs very hard selling in the Third World. So far, there has been heavy concentration on the national development rationale emphasizing the adverse social and economic consequences of high fertility, and the potential social and economic benefits of family planning.

The health rationale for family planning

The major proposition in this chapter is that, while not undermining the social and economic argument for family planning, the health benefits of family planning seem to be of more direct relevance to families, communities and whole nations.

There can be little doubt that impressive health benefits result from adequate spacing of pregnancy, limiting the number of siblings, and appropriate timing of pregnancy in relation to the age of the mother. It has been estimated, for instance, that adequate and universal family planning in the United States alone can result in a 29% reduction of infant mortality. The impact in countries with higher child mortality may be even greater. Similarly, the protection of mothers' health and securing their survival can accrue from appropriate planning of pregnancy. It has been estimated that if one form of high risk pregnancy, that is, pregnancy after age 35, is avoided in Thailand, the life of approximately 1500 women would be saved every year.

A similar saving of life would result from avoided teenage pregnancy or postponing the first child until after age 18, or better still, after age 20.

In Africa, adequate spacing of children would virtually eliminate a disease called kwashiorkor, which is the African interpretation for 'the disease of the deposed child'. This is a case of protein-calorie malnutrition that affects a child who is on breast milk and whose mother gets a new pregnancy. She may stop lactating him altogether, or her milk may become less adequate, being shared by two organisms. The infant becomes so deprived of nutrition that his pitch-black hair loses its colour and becomes dirty reddish, due to a lack of protein needed to maintain the original health colour and texture of the hair.

Likewise, rupture of the uterus, an obstetric condition, now common in the Third World, would virtually disappear if the number of pregnancies were limited. The condition is basically due to repeated stretching of the uterine wall with repeated pregnancies to the extent that in a later pregnancy the wall thins out so much that it explodes. This condition is now extremely rare in low parity regions.

In the following discussion, a systematic approach to characterize the health aspects of family planning is provided as a basis for endorsing the health rationale for family planning. In this discussion, eight major areas of family planning and health will be considered.

FAMILY PLANNING AND CHILD HEALTH

World experience indicates that pregnancies that are too many (high parity or birth order), or closely spaced (at short birth intervals), or occurring too early (teenage pregnancy), or too late (after age 35) are associated with increased health risks to the fetus, infant and young child. Scientists usually measure these risks in terms of the proportion of pregnancies that do not reach term (fetal loss), babies born dead (stillbirths), or of low birth weight (premature), the proportion of infants who die within the first year of life (infant mortality), the proportion of children dying before age 5 (pre-school or child mortality), or the increased frequency of disease (morbidity).

Parity and birth order effect

The chances of survival are relatively better for earlier born children than for later born children, with the exception of the firstborn child who usually sustains a slightly higher risk especially for teenage mothers. A study from India of 1000 consecutive births indicate that the risk of mortality before or immediately after birth was 13% for firstborn children, 5% for second born, 11% for third, fourth and fifth born, 16% for sixth through ninth born, and 25% for tenth and later born children. Similar results were reported from both developing and industrialized countries including a WHO sponsored collaborative study in ten Asian, African and Latin American countries.

The question of whether this phenomenon is common to both rich and poor classes was answered by a nationwide study in England and Wales, which included all births during one year (Figure 1). The risk of infant mortality for comparable birth orders was shown to be higher for infants of low social class than for those of higher social class, a not unexpected finding. However, the study also demonstrated that the risks of mortality increased almost progressively with birth order. Thus, the benefits of family planning are by no means limited to the poor.

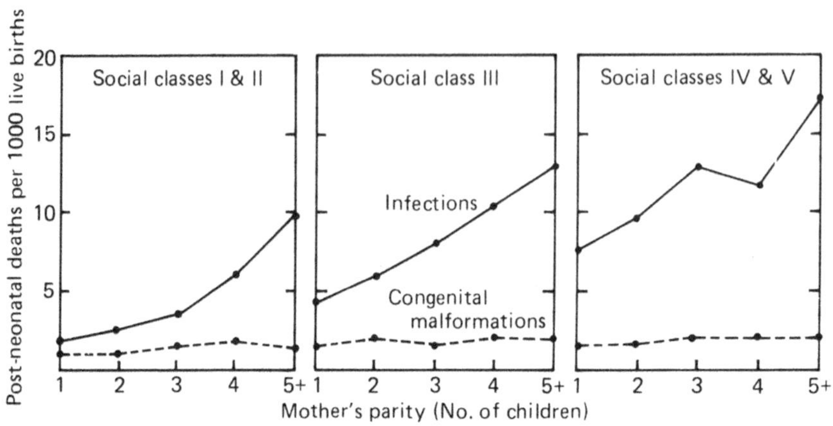

Figure 1 Postneonatal mortality from infections and congenital malformations

Effect of birth interval

Pregnancies occurring at short intervals, especially those occurring at less than 1 year of a previous one, carry greater risks of ending up in fetal loss, stillbirth, premature babies, and infant and child mortality. These risks are still fairly high for intervals of less than 2 years. This is because adequate time is needed for the reproductive system of the mother to recover from pregnancy and childbirth, and for her body in general to build up its depleted reserves in preparation for another pregnancy. Successive pregnancies are the usual pattern in less developed countries where the problem is compounded further by widespread undernutrition of mothers. This will affect not only the outcome of pregnancy, but also the nutritional status of the child already born whose main source of good protein is his mother's milk, but also the newcomer since both have to share the limited nutritional resources of an overtaxed mother. Reference already has been made to kwashiorkor, a disease in lactating children whose mothers are pregnant with another child, which is prevalent in Africa and also common in other developing countries.

Timing of pregnancy

Sensible reproductive planning requires not only limiting and spacing pregnancies, but also proper timing to maternal ages with minimal risks. For the age at which conception occurs may determine whether the pregnancy will come successfully to term, whether the child born alive will survive the risks of infancy and childhood, and whether or not he or she will be the victim of disabling, handicapping conditions. The risks are greater for pregnancies occurring under age 18 and at age 35 or later. For instance, the risk of fetal loss, prematurity and child mortality is much greater at these age extremes than for ages 20–30, the safest age span for human reproduction. Mongolism or mental retardation increases 20 or more times for children born to older mothers (age 35 or later).

Health risks to survivors

Children who happen to survive the mortality hazards of unplanned pregnancies appear to be more likely to suffer from a variety of diseases, disabilities, and chronic ill-health than their counterparts in planned families. Such survivors are more prone to infectious diseases, malnutrition and stunted growth and development.

Effect on intellectual development

It is alarming that the intellectual development of children of high birth orders or in large families is typically much lower than that of children of low birth order or smaller families. Intelligence is usually measured in terms of intelligent quotient or IQ. Surveys in more and less developed countries confirm that the IQ level, on the average, starts to drop in the fourth, fifth, and later born children (Figures 2 and 3). Furthermore, manifest mental retardation is more common among children from large than small families. Among the possible factors influencing lower intelligence in later born children are the declining parental interest, and decreased verbal and supportive contact with a child in a large family.

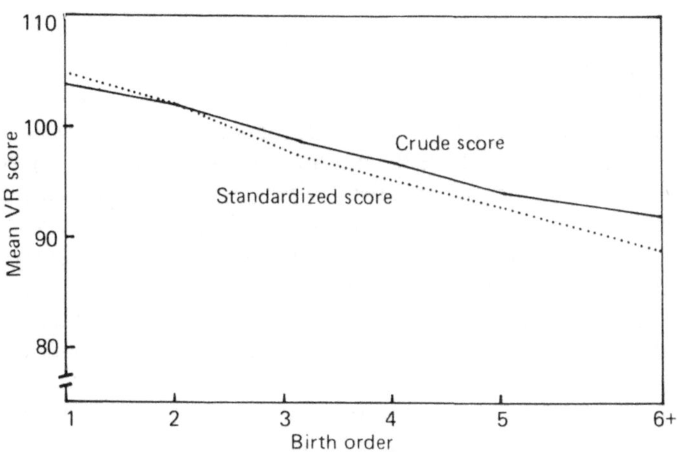

Figure 2 Relation of verbal reasoning (VR) score to birth order

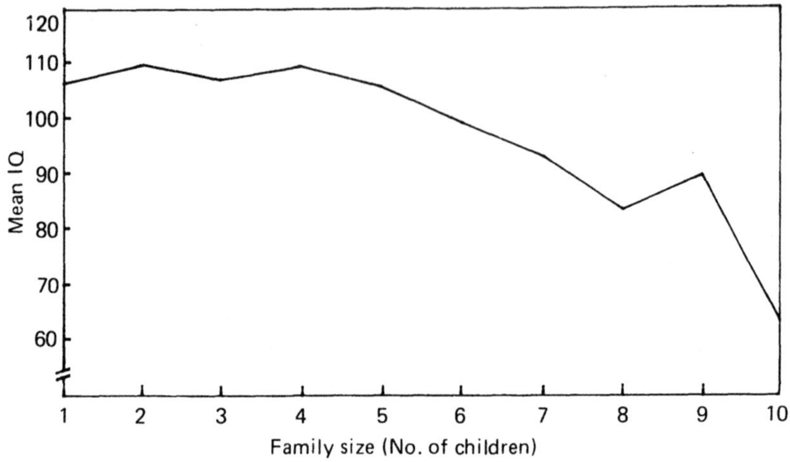

Figure 3 Size of family compared with mean IQ of children

FAMILY PLANNING AND MATERNAL HEALTH

A mother producing children under unfavourable family formation circumstances is also at a higher risk of mortality and disease, of complications of pregnancy and difficult labour.

Increased maternal mortality

Women with large numbers of births, commonly termed by gynaecologists and obstetricians as multiparas (with three or more children), or grand multiparas (with six or more children) are themselves at a higher risk of death from diseases associated with pregnancy, labour, and puerperium. Women with six or more children have three or four times the risk of dying compared to women with one or two children. This high maternal mortality is due to the rupture of the uterus (from repeated stretching), hypertension, kidney diseases, or haemorrhage associated with placental abnormalities. Another factor affecting maternal mortality is maternal age. Mothers who conceive between the ages of 30–40 have twice the risk of dying in pregnancy or childbirth as women aged 20–30, the prime years for childbearing. For women over age 40, the risk increases progressively to four or five times that of women aged 20–30. There is also an increased risk for women conceiving under age 20 as will be discussed under teenage pregnancy. Thus, the risk of maternal mortality in relation to age describes a curve that looks like the

letter J, with relatively high risks under age 20, lowest risks between 20–30, and progressively increasing risks after 30 (Figure 4). Medically speaking, pregnancy after age 30 and, decidedly after age 35, are considered 'high risk pregnancies' that should be avoided.

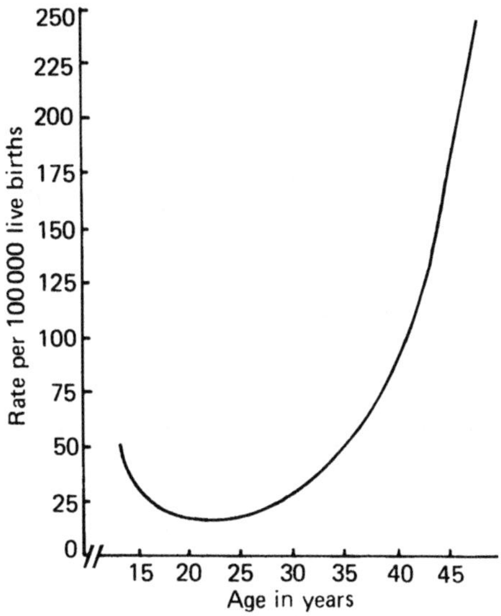

Figure 4 Maternal mortality (US). From Judith S. Mausner and Anita K. Bahn (1974). *Epidemiology: An Introductory Text* (Philadelphia: W. B. Saunders Co.), with permission of authors and publishers

Increased obstetric risks

Besides mortality, pregnancies to high parity mothers (multiparas) are associated with higher incidence of pregnancy complications and difficult labour. Included are toxaemias of pregnancy, hypertension, anaemia of pregnancy, placental abnormalities, malpresentation of fetus (e.g. breech or limb presentation), and haemorrhage. There is also an increased risk of uterine inertia (lazy uterus) and rupture of the uterus.

Increased non-obstetric conditions

High parity is also associated with increased risk of prolapse, cancer of the cervix, diabetes, and rheumatiod arthritis. Studies in England and the US, for example, have shown a definite rise of the occurrence of diabetes with parity (Figure 5).

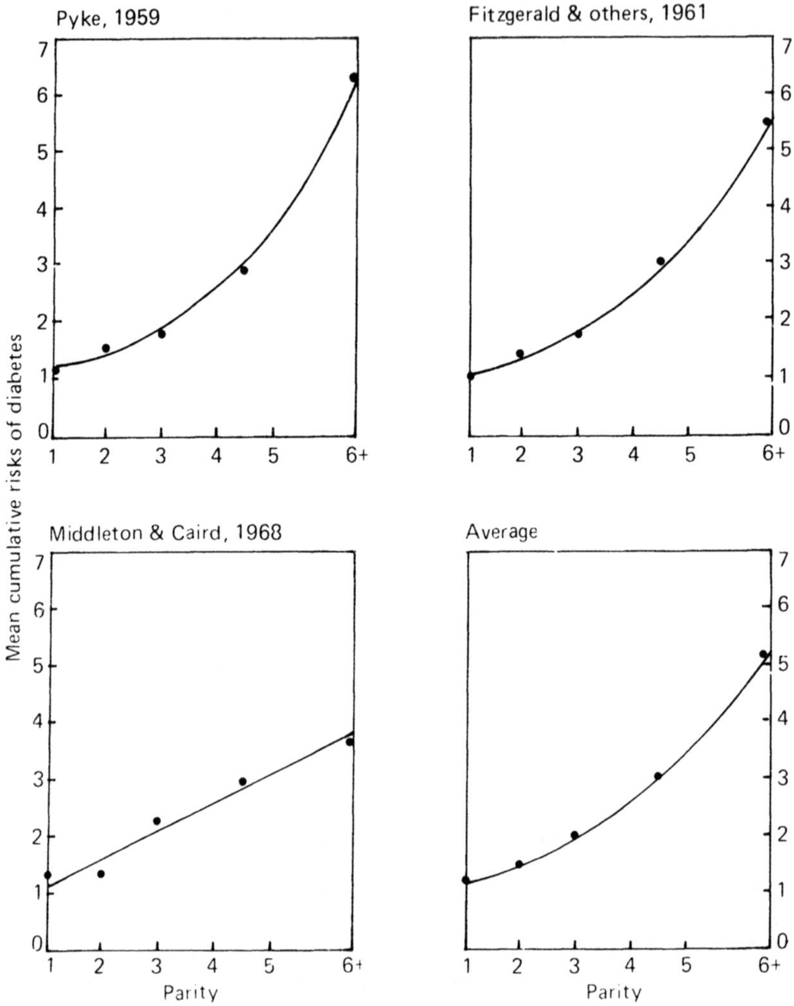

Figure 5 Mean cumulative risks of diabetes at ages 50 to 80 years, relative to nulliparae (=1), England

FAMILY PLANNING AND TEENAGE PREGNANCY

Teenage childbearing is a serious health, social, and psychological problem that has reached epidemic proportions in many countries, both developed and less developed. The problem is compounded when births are out of wedlock or when induced abortion is resorted to.

The problem of rising teenage pregnancy

Some 10–15% of all births in the world, that is, approximately 12–18 million births a year, occur to teenage mothers. The problem is not restricted to the less developed societies where marriage (usually arranged marriages) occur at extremely young ages, and where teenage contraception is non-existent. The problem of teenage pregnancy is increasing even in the more developed countries where almost one in every five or six pregnancies occurs to a teenager. In the United States, about 10% of all teenagers get pregnant every year; one third of these pregnancies are out of wedlock. In East Germany, 23% of all births in 1972 occurred to teenage girls.

Health hazards of teenage pregnancy

Reference has already been made to the increased risk of maternal mortality with a teenage pregnancy which is usually more prone to toxaemia, anaemia, and difficult labour. In addition, offspring of teenagers are more prone to die in infancy, to have low birth weight, or have higher risks of congenital anomalies. Compared to a pregnancy at age 20–24, for example:

* maternal mortality risk is 60% higher for teenagers;
* babies of young teens are two to three times more likely to die in the first year of life;
* the risk of low birth weight is twice as high for infants of teenagers.

FAMILY PLANNING METHODS AND HEALTH

In recent decades, the use of contraceptive methods, abortion, and sterilization have substantially increased. Never before have so many people used drugs, devices, and surgery to control their fertility. The health aspects of fertility control measures warrant careful consideration.

There is increasing debate about the safety of fertility control methods, especially the Pill. Intensive studies show increased risks of certain health conditions with the use of the Pill, especially by women over age 35. Included in these hazards are hypertension, thromboembolic phenomena, and liver and gall bladder disease, to mention only a few. It should, however, be pointed out that these hazards are extremely rare and that the risks of the Pill's side effects are much lower than the risks of the pregnancies they prevent. For example, the excess mortality of thromboembolism in England associated with pill use is one eighth the risk of pregnancy (0.00003 for the Pill compared to

0.00025 for pregnancy). Other contraceptives have non-fatal complications – the IUD is associated with blood loss and backache. Abortion, when performed illegally under unsanitary conditions is associated with increased health hazards of haemorrhage, infection, and mortality. Medical abortion, however, especially in the first trimester is relatively safe. Sterilization is safe in the male, while the risks of female sterilization have been on the decline with the use of new methods not requiring general anaesthesia.

There are also some other benefits of contraceptives. Besides avoiding the social and psychological trauma of unwanted pregnancies, certain contraceptives have benefits: the diaphragm and condom protect against cancer of the cervix, the condom is a preventive measure against venereal diseases, and the Pill is associated with a lower incidence of benign tumours of the breast.

Nevertheless, the search for safer contraceptives should continue and should receive the utmost priority by research and donor agencies.

LACTATION AND HEALTH

Lactation used to be the main method of feeding a child until it was almost replaced by artificial feeding especially in the more developed countries and by liberated women. The health aspects of lactation are currently under scrutiny.

Since this subject is discussed in more detail in Chapter 3, only a brief note is necessary here. Recent research has brought back confidence in the health benefits of lactation, a confidence that was for a while lost in the increasing publicity tide of artificial feeding. Lactation, during the early period of life and later with supplements, is the best source for nutrients to the infant. As a concern in the family planning context, there are a few important statements.

(a) Prolonged lactation may have some contraceptive value through prolonging postpartum amenorrhoea. This is, however, a debatable issue. Research is needed to determine the amount of contraceptive protection that lactation confers to a woman under different circumstances, and independently of abstinence and lower exposure to pregnancy during lactation in certain cultures.

(b) Hormonal contraceptives, particularly the Pill, may lower the nutritional quality of milk. This is of concern in poor families where mother's milk is the main source of high quality protein and other nutrients for the baby.

(c) Child survival prolongs birth interval perhaps through prolonged lactation and postpartum amenorrhoea as compared, for example, with intervals following stillbirth or early infant death.

FAMILY PLANNING AND INFERTILITY

A discussion of family planning and health can never be complete without a consideration of infertility.

From a health viewpoint, family planning should encompass the prevention and treatment of infertility and subfecundity, especially if these occur involuntarily before the achievement of desired family size. Infertility, especially in certain societal and cultural settings, can be a tragic problem affecting the physical, social and mental wellbeing of married couples. In certain cultures, a woman's status and family status are related to having children, preferably sons.

The prevalence of infertility varies from place to place, and from time to time. It is estimated that about 10–15% of married couples are unable to conceive, and the prevalence is higher in certain localities, particularly sub-Saharan Africa. Infertility should not however be confused with childlessness which may be due to inability to conceive (infertility proper), inability to bring a pregnancy to term (fetal loss and habitual abortion), and inability to keep a child alive (child loss). Childlessness may thus be as high as 30%, that is, about one in every three woman of childbearing age may have no children in certain communities. Thus, if infertility and childlessness are used interchangeably, the figures are greatly inflated.

Nevertheless, the management of infertility problems should be incorporated in family planning services, even in overpopulated countries. This would 'ironically' increase the acceptability of family planning since it would demonstrate that such a programme is for the welfare of the people.

FAMILY PLANNING AND HEALTH DELIVERY SYSTEMS

A burning question to policy-makers is whether or not to integrate family planning services into health services. There are arguments on both sides of this vital issue.

There is increasing inclination to integrate family planning into health services. In general, family planning services stand to benefit from the long experience of the health professionals in providing preventive and curative services. Not only will the development and implementation of family planning services benefit from the methods used in developing and implementing health programmes, but also family planning research and evaluation will benefit from the health service research techniques. Opponents to integration argue that the use of health service research and implementation methods can be made without the necessity of integration.

To be more specific, proponents of integration argue that:

(a) Integration would maximize the service components and guarantee the most efficient use of available supplies, equipment, transportation, telecommunication, personnel and organizational structure. Integrated health and family planning services would have greater appeal to families who prefer to seek a single source of care for their multiple health problems.

(b) In many conservative cultures, there is an obvious reluctance to be seen in a family planning clinic. Appearance at a general health clinic where diversified services are offered would not carry the same stigma.

(c) Many family planning services have suffered from inadequate follow-up of acceptors. This could be avoided by developing follow-up services in conjunction with other health care services.

(d) Family planning services can also be provided as a routine part of prenatal, postpartum, and postabortion programmes; child health care; immunization programmes; and other family health services. The rationale for this approach is psychological as well as operational since it would introduce mothers and families to family planning services at the time of highest motivation.

(e) Certain family planning methods, particularly IUD insertions, hormonal contraception, and surgical methods, require medical training in regard to case selection, implementation, follow-up, and management of side-effects. Backup support by the medical community and health teams is highly desirable.

(f) The support of the medical profession for family planning efforts has been crucial in gaining political and cultural acceptance of the programme. This support is always required, regardless of whether or not the family planning programme is integrated into health services.

Opponents to integration and even some proponents of it as well, warn strongly that in certain countries or settings, integration of family planning into health services may hinder rather than enhance programme effectiveness. This is because:

1. The coverage of health services in many developing countries is often a meagre 10%, especially in rural areas. This is hardly enough for the family planning targets.

2. Health services tend to be over-concentrated in urban areas, while excessive fertility, with its attendant health problems, is highest in rural areas.

3. Health services in developing countries have so far been orientated toward providing services for those who seek them, while in family planning the burden of motivating the clientele to seek services is on the programme itself.

4. Health services in the developing world are visibly overburdened, and family planning may be considered an additional burden. Certainly the health

authorities would not give family planning a priority higher than that of other pressing health problems.

IMPACT OF CHILD LOSS ON FERTILITY LEVEL

An important question that is being considered by students of family planning and demography is whether or not child loss experience can affect fertility levels of families and societies.

So far we have been discussing the impact of unplanned fertility (including high fertility) on health (including child mortality). There is evidence to indicate that the reverse may occur under certain societal, biological, and cultural circumstances. In other words, while high fertility may result in high child mortality, likewise, child loss experience may result in high fertility. This can occur in different ways which may explain this peculiar relationship.

(a) In absence of contraception, the birth interval after a child loss is usually shorter than when the child survives. This is because of the cessation of lactation which is believed to have some contraceptive effect, either by itself (biological) or through abstinence and decreased frequency of intercourse (behavioural). In this way, child loss affects higher fertility through involuntary mechanisms.

(b) Couples who lose one or more of their children will be more inclined to compensate for the loss by having additional children. This is particularly so when a male child is lost and is called *replacement mechanism.*

(c) Couples may not have lost a child, themselves, but they are living in an area where child loss is high. Hence, they have as many children as they can so that they can insure enough of them survive. This is called *insurance mechanism,* and is highly relevant in developing countries where for centuries child mortality has been extremely high and in response, fertility was kept high.

(d) Another mechanism may be imposed by the society where the norm is to have large numbers of children, especially sons. This is the *societal mechanism.*

Under these circumstances, fertility is kept high and acceptance of family planning is minimal. That this actually exists has been proven by many studies, including the WHO collaborative study in three continents. One of the findings of the study is that couples who lost children early in their reproductive life were reluctant to accept family planning, compared to couples with no child loss who were more prone to accept and use contraception.

Based on this type of evidence, a hypothesis is usually proposed denoting that couples will continue to resist family planning until they are assured of improved child survival. Hence, policymakers are now convinced that programmes to reduce child mortality should go hand in hand with family planning.

THE ACCEPTABILITY OF THE HEALTH RATIONALE FOR FAMILY PLANNING

It is becoming increasingly evident that promoting family planning for demographic reasons is doomed to failure in many areas especially in Africa, the Middle East, and the Muslim communities in general. Planning the family for health benefits is, on the other hand, more acceptable to many conservative cultures and for countries where overpopulation is matched by adequate resources. A prominent example is that the Islamic doctrine has always accepted family planning for health reasons. The Quran itself says: 'mothers shall beget no harm from bearing children'
All the *fatuas* (religious opinion) given by Muslim leaders endorse avoiding pregnancy if it would result in health risks to the mother in particular. In the same vein, Islam promotes lactation and spacing. The Prophet Mohammad has particularly warned against conception while a woman is still lactating another child. He called that practice *al-ghail,* and indicated that it would have long lasting effect on the health of a child.

The acceptability of the health theme for family planning to the medical profession should also be considered. For, even though the responsibility for family planning lies mainly with parents, it also lies with the medical profession and health organizations who must further these ideas through education, health services planning, and daily professional practice.

CONCLUSIONS

Health safeguards for human reproduction

World-wide experience indicates that effective family planning can favourably influence the health, development, and wellbeing of families and individual family members. Considering the three major variables in family formation, namely parity, birth interval, and timing, there are safe landmarks for human reproduction summarized in Figure 6, which is based on the world-wide

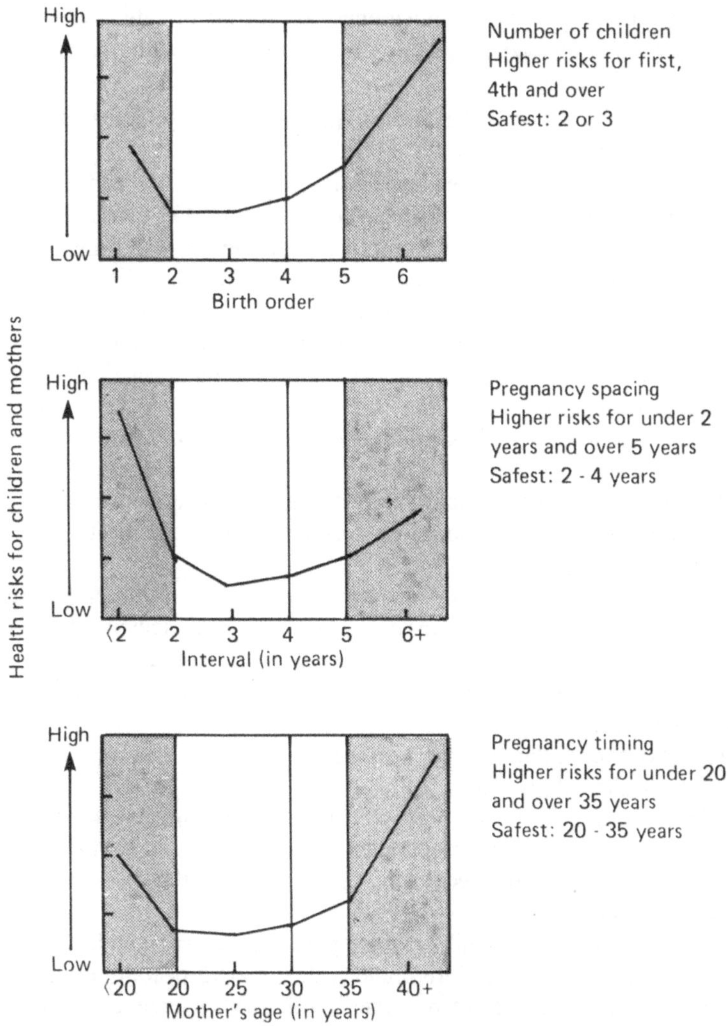

Figure 6 Safe landmarks for human reproduction

experience in this regard. In drawing up a healthy reproductive plan, parents and policy-makers should observe the following rules of thumb in regard to relative safety:

1. The *optimal age* for having children is between the ages of 20–29 or 20–35. With a pregnancy at younger or older ages, there is a risk of disease, disability or death for both mother and child. This means that age at marriage may wisely be raised to 20 (if possible) for girls, and more importantly, that

the first pregnancy should be postponed to age 20 or later because of the confirmed risks of teenage pregnancy. It also means avoiding pregnancy after age 35.

2. The *interval* between the end of one pregnancy and the beginning of another should be no less than 2 years.

3. Two or three children, well spaced, properly timed, and expressly wanted are the best number from a health viewpoint. Health risks increase for fourth, fifth, and later children, and for unwanted children of any order.

4. To minimize the relatively high risk (which often is difficult to eliminate altogether) for the first child, the first pregnancy should not occur below age 20. The mother should be in adequate health and nutritional status, and should receive proper and early prenatal and paranatal medical care.

5. Breast feeding should be the rule for every child, to be supplemented by other foods under medical guidance. By no means should a lactating woman conceive.

6. Contraception should take precedence to abortion. However, when abortion is unavoidable, it should be performed under the best medical and aseptic conditions.

7. The pill should be totally avoided after age 40 (and preferably 35), when another method should be used. Couples who have achieved their desired family size should be advised to consider male or female sterilization.

8. Management of infertility should become an integral part of family planning services.

9. Genetic counselling should also be incorporated into family planning and family health education.

To close with an optimistic note, we might report that the World Medical Society (a society of all the national medical associations in the world) has adopted, in its Stockholm meeting in 1974, a proposition submitted by this author, which says that:

> 'The prescription of family planning will reduce substantial health risks to mothers and children, and hence, should become a part of routine patient care for responsible health professionals everywhere in the world.'

Bibliography

Nortman, D. (1974). Parental age as a factor in pregnancy outcome and child development. *Reports on Population and Family Planning.* (New York: The Population Council)

Omran, A. R. (1971). *The Health Theme in Family Planning.* Monograph 16. (Chapel Hill: The Carolina Population Center)

Omran, A. R. and Standley, C. C. (eds.) (1976). *Family Formation Patterns and*

Health. (Geneva: World Health Association)
Omran, A. R. and Omran, K. F. (1977). Family planning and health, the vital connection. In Gardener *et al.* (eds.) ***Village and Household Availability of Contraceptives.*** (Seattle: Battelle)
Tietze, C., Bongaarts, J. and Shearer, B. (1976). Mortality associated with control of fertility. *Family Planning Perspectives,* **8,** 6

3

Fertility and lactation

Jeroen van Ginneken

INTRODUCTION	38
INCIDENCE AND DURATION OF LACTATION	38
Full and partial lactation	40
Postpartum abstinence and lactation	40
LACTATION AND BIRTH INTERVALS	41
Pregnancy rates before and after return of menstruation	42
LACTATION AND AMENORRHOEA	43
Limitations of lactation in extending amenorrhoea	44
DECLINE OF LACTATION AND ITS CONSEQUENCES	45
Consequences for infant mortality and morbidity	46
Consequences for fertility	46
Measures to protect breast feeding	47
LACTATION AND MODERN CONTRACEPTION	48
Limitations of breast feeding as a birth spacing method	49
Choice of contraceptive methods and time of introduction	50
CONCLUSIONS	51

INTRODUCTION

Many mothers in rural areas of developing countries nurse their babies for 1–2 years after delivery. They believe that breast feeding is good for the health of their child. In order to be able to nurse for a long time, mothers know that they should not become pregnant too quickly after birth and that an adequate birth interval is required. Usually, women are aware that prolonged lactation has the capacity to postpone the next pregnancy and that adequate birth spacing can be achieved by means of this practice. They also know, however, that one cannot rely on this method indefinitely and that another pregnancy is likely to occur sooner or later. Indeed, many mothers will continue to nurse until or after the next pregnancy occurs.

In several developing countries, spacing between births is achieved by lactation together with abstinence from sexual relations. Abstinence after delivery is practised in such societies to make sure that lactation continues for 1–2 years and is not interrupted by another pregnancy. Abstinence is often reinforced by the belief that intercourse before weaning is dangerous for the child as it poisons the mother's milk, or reduces the supply of milk. Due to prolonged breast feeding, with or without the support of post partum abstinence, birth intervals in rural areas of many developing countries range from 30 to 36 months. Such intervals are achieved in the absence of modern contraception and an important question that arises is – to what extent can modern family planning programmes take advantage of the existence of these traditional birth spacing methods?

INCIDENCE AND DURATION OF LACTATION

Table 1 shows percentages of women who started breast feeding after birth, together with mean duration of breast feeding (among those who practised it). The studies represented in Table 1 have been conducted since 1967 and the sample size included at least 500 women or births. Some of the nationwide data were derived from recently completed reports of the World Fertility Survey.

Lactation is nearly universal in rural areas of low income countries for which data are shown, with the exception of Chile. The percentages of women who initiate nursing in urban areas are somewhat smaller than in rural areas – a result which is consistent with many other surveys. The mean duration of lactation varies considerably. Nursing lasts for 1–2 years in most countries that were surveyed and there is a tendency for women in rural areas to nurse longer than those in urban areas. Women tend to nurse for shorter periods in countries in South and Middle America as compared to other regions.

TABLE 1 Incidence and duration of lactation in selected countries

Residence Region and country	*Urban/rural*	*Per cent starting lactation*	*Mean duration of lactation (for women who started) (in months)*
Africa			
Algeria	u/r	90–95	17.5
Kenya	u/r	97	14.5
Nigeria	r	95–100	22
Senegal	r	95–100	24
Upper Volta	r	95–100	17.5
Zaire	r	95–100	22
South and Middle America			
Chile	r	68	6
Colombia	u	79	5.5
Dominican Republic	u/r	90	10
Guatemala	r	—	18
Martinique	u/r	93	10
Venezuela	u	84	7.5
Asia			
Fiji	u/r	—	8.5
India, Calcutta	u	93	16.5
India, Tamil Nadu	r	98	22
Indonesia	r	99	25.5
Malaysia	u/r	81	9
Philippines	u	76	10
Sri Lanka	u/r	95	18.5
South Korea	u/r	94	20.5
Taiwan	u/r	93	16
Thailand	u	86	12
Turkey	u	95	13

Prolonged breast feeding is, in general, much more common and practised for a longer period of time in low income countries than in high income countries. On the basis of two surveys conducted in France five years ago and in Great Britain 10 years ago, it is estimated that about half the women began breast feeding, but only continued for an average of one and two months respectively.

Full and partial lactation

Mothers usually start with full breast feeding when the infant receives no other supplements. After some months there is a gradual change to partial breast feeding when solid foods and/or animal milk are added to the baby's diet. A few surveys give information about the length of full breast feeding in comparison to partial breast feeding. In a rural area of Nigeria, the median duration of full lactation was found to be 11 months, while the median duration of full lactation and partial lactation was 15 months. In the Punjab, India, full lactation was practised for six out of 21 months (median) and in rural Bangladesh it was nine out of 25 months. On the other hand, in a rural area in Zaire supplementary feeding was introduced after an average of 3 months, but the women continued breast feeding for nearly 2 years. In Manila, Philippines, supplementary feeding was introduced in the second month (on average).

These figures show that the period of time during which full breast feeding is practised varies considerably. From a nutritional point of view, it is recommended that the child should rely exclusively on breast milk for a period of 4–6 months after birth. Solid foods should be gradually introduced around that time and breast milk should continue to be given for at least 1 and preferably 2 years as a supplement after birth. A comparison of the figures cited above with these nutritional requirements indicates that there are areas where full breast feeding continues too long and probably results in an increased incidence of nutritional and other disorders. It is also clear that, in particular in urban areas, supplementary feeding is introduced too early.

Postpartum abstinence and lactation

Until recently, information on postpartum abstinence was derived from anthropological sources. However, during the past decade, data have also become available from a number of surveys conducted on breast feeding and related topics. These surveys show that postpartum abstinence is practised for an average of between 18 to 24 months in a number of African countries, such as Ghana, Nigeria, Upper Volta and Zaire. In these countries the duration of abstinence is as long as, or even exceeds, the duration of lactation. Considerable variation in this practice was found within Africa. For instance, in some rural areas of Central Africa, the practice is unknown while in other parts it is quite common. Considerable variation exists by residence: abstinence is practised for a longer time in rural areas than in urban areas.

Less is known about the situation in Asia and in Latin America. A number of studies in India have found an average duration of abstinence of 5–6 months after birth. Abstinence is often achieved by the socially accepted custom whereby women return to the parents' home for several months after a delivery. Prolonged abstinence of about 2 years after birth is practised in some rural areas of Indonesia, which is as long as the period of lactation. Again, however, large variations in abstinence are found within rural areas of that country. It is likely that the practice of postpartum abstinence exists in various other areas of Asia and Latin America, but its duration is much shorter than that of lactation.

LACTATION AND BIRTH INTERVALS

Average birth intervals of nursing mothers who had weaned their children are compared in Figure 1 with those of mothers who had not nursed because of fetal deaths, still births, or other reasons. This figure shows such intervals in six selected studies populations who either did not use contraception or only used it to a small extent. Average birth intervals were substantially longer for nursing than for non-nursing women. The difference ranges from 15 to 19 months in Bangladesh, Nigeria, and Senegal to 7 months in Taiwan. These survey results suggest that lactation lengthens birth intervals substantially. It

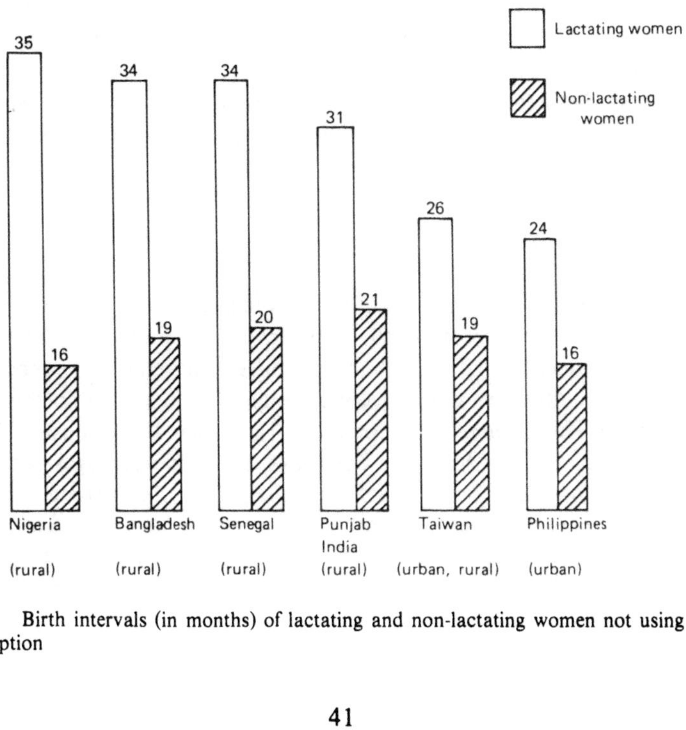

Figure 1 Birth intervals (in months) of lactating and non-lactating women not using modern contraception

should be added that the duration of lactation averaged about two years in rural areas of Bangladesh, Nigeria, Senegal and Punjab (India) in which these studies were undertaken, 16 months in Taiwan and 10 months in the Philippines.

The data of Figure 1 should be interpreted with caution because several factors were not adequately controlled. One of these is the extent of malnutrition in the study populations. Malnutrition may have had an impact on amenorrhoea independent of the impact of lactation. Other factors may have been the practice of abstinence from sexual relations after birth, or the frequency of such sexual relations. One can estimate the effect of lactation on birth intervals by determining first how much longer the birth intervals are for nursing than for non-nursing women. Next, one can calculate to what extent this difference contributes to average birth intervals. In rural Bangladesh, for instance, birth intervals averaged about 36 months, while these intervals were increased by 15 months by lactation, which means an effect of 15/36 or 42%.

Similarly, on the basis of data obtained in a survey in Nigeria it was estimated that lactation was responsible for a reduction in fertility of 32%. In view of the fact that abstinence exceeded the duration of lactation in that society, fertility would have been 45% higher in the absence of post-natal abstinence. In many other low income countries, this impact on birth intervals is smaller than in rural Bangladesh and Nigeria. In Taiwan, for example, where birth intervals were about 30 months, lactation prolonged birth intervals by 7 months – an effect of 23%. It is clear from these calculations that the impact of lactation (and abstinence) on fertility levels in many countries is substantial. It is estimated that in most low income countries lactation reduces fertility up to 25%.

Pregnancy rates before and after return of menstruation

Ovulation is followed by menstruation if fertilization does not take place, but menstruation can also occur in the absence of ovulation. It is important to know to what extent pregnancies occur before resumption of menstruation. Results of five studies using prospective designs are available on this subject. These studies, which have been conducted in India, Bangladesh, Chile, the Philippines and USA (Alaskan Eskimos) show percentages of women conceiving during amenorrhoea of 7.0, 6.8, 7.0, 2.5 and 2.6 per cent respectively. Several other studies have reported on the incidence of pregnancies during amenorrhoea, but these have not been used, either because data were collected by retrospective studies, or because there were indications that proportions of women had stopped nursing before becoming pregnant or were using contraception.

A few studies have also determined pregnancy rates for nursing and non-nursing women after resumption of menstruation. The results of these studies were contradictory. Two studies found no significant differences in the rate of conception after resumption of menstruation between nursing and non-nursing women. However, two other studies concluded that nursing women conceived on an average 3–4 months later after resumption of menstruation as compared to non-nursing women.

LACTATION AND AMENORRHOEA

From a physiological point of view, lactation postpones the next pregnancy by inhibiting ovulation and by delaying resumption of the menstrual cycle. Suckling of the infant is important for this suppression of the menstrual cycle, because suckling leads to the release of prolactin which not only plays an important role in milk production, but also inhibits the release of gonadotrophins which initiate resumption of the menstrual cycle. Data on the effect of lactation on postpartum amenorrhoea derived from 9 selected surveys are provided in Figure 2.

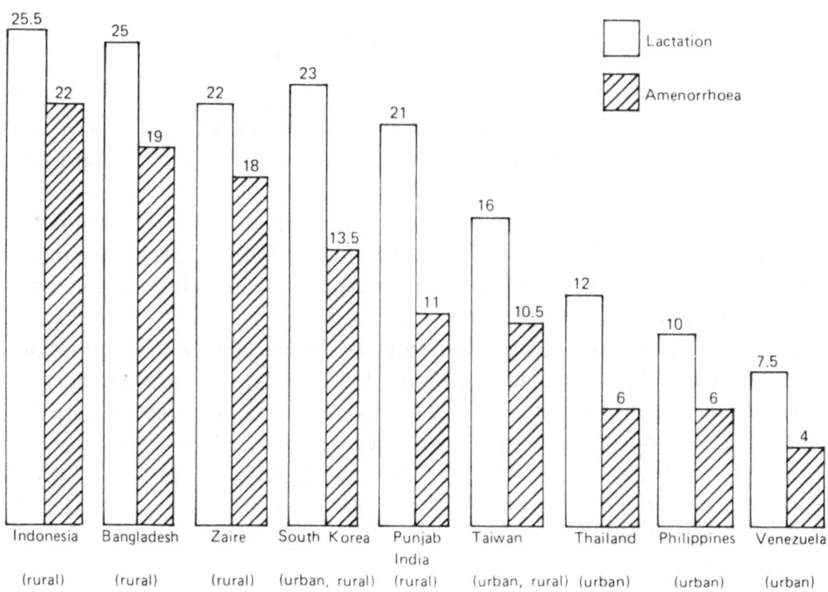

Figure 2 Mean duration of lactation and postpartum amenorrhoea (in months) among women who had weaned their infants

This figure shows that the practice of nursing can have a substantial effect on the duration of amenorrhoea. Duration of lactation was about 2 years on average in rural areas of Zaire, Indonesia and Bangladesh, whereas duration of amenorrhoea ranged from 18 to 22 months. On the other hand, in urban areas in Thailand, the Philippines and Venezuela, duration of lactation ranged from 7.5 to 12 months, whereas periods of amenorrhoea lasted from 4 to 6 months. Various studies have shown that the period of postpartum amenorrhoea averaged about 2 to 3 months for non-nursing women and the impact of lactation alone on amenorrhoea is, therefore, about 2 to 3 months less than the periods of amenorrhoea shown in Figure 2. The practice of prolonged breast feeding can, therefore, lengthen the period of amenorrhoea ranging from a maximum of 18 months (in rural areas of Zaire, Indonesia and Bangladesh) to a minimum of about 2 months (in urban areas of Venezuela). It has been observed that in some rural areas women spend from 30 to 40% of their reproductive years in amenorrhoea and this implies a substantial reduction in fertility. The long intervals of amenorrhoea observed in rural areas of Zaire, Indonesia and Bangladesh were probably the combined effect of lactation and some degree of malnutrition in the mother.

Limitations of lactation in extending amenorrhoea

Another finding is that lactation cannot postpone the resumption of menses indefinitely. In a nationwide survey of a healthy population in Taiwan, it was observed that the longer lactation lasted, the less it added to the average duration of amenorrhoea. In other words, the longer lactation lasted, the more likely it was for menses to return. The maximum duration of amenorrhoea observed was about 15 months for women nursing between 30 and 36 months. In women below 30 years of age, the duration of amenorrhoea levelled off to about 12–13 months as the maximum.

Another important aspect to consider is the variability of resumption of menses. Although a median duration of 12 months of amenorrhoea was observed in studies in India, Taiwan and South Korea (see Figure 2), a considerable proportion of nursing women experienced resumption of menstruation much earlier or later than that average. These surveys show, for instance, that among women who had weaned their children, 14–19% had resumed menses within 3 months after delivery. On aggregate, prolonged lactation exercised a considerable impact on amenorrhoea, but for nearly one-fifth of the women this was not the case. This variability in return of menses is very likely related to the fact that women change from full to partial lactation at different intervals after birth. It has been found that menstruation (and ovulation) return much earlier in women who give supplementary foods to their infants, than in women who are providing breast-milk only. These changes from full to partial lactation explain in part why resumption of menstruation can occur quite early after birth. During partial lactation, the amount of suckling by the baby is much less intensive than during full breast feeding. This affects the hormonal changes which initiate resumption of the menstrual cycle.

DECLINE OF LACTATION AND ITS CONSEQUENCES

In many low income countries, particularly in urban areas, breast feeding has declined rapidly and has been replaced by bottle feeding. Two examples will illustrate this decline. In Singapore, the percentage of low income women who were breast feeding three months after birth decreased from nearly 80% in 1951 to 10% in 1971. In some cities in Southern Brazil, similar declines were observed at 6 months after birth – from 68% in 1940 to 12% in 1974.

This decrease in incidence and duration of breast feeding is related to a number of 'modernization' processes:

* widespread use of advertising techniques to promote infant formulas;
* negative attitudes towards breast feeding by physicians and nurses in health services (in particular hospitals);
* employment of mothers outside the home which is generally incompatible with frequent nursing;
* absence in nuclear families of relatives who have experience with nursing;
* adoption of attitudes in which breasts are felt to have an exclusive aesthetic and erotic role;
* convenience of bottle feeding in relation to greater liberation of mothers for activities outside the home.

The influence of some of these modernization processes can be inferred from survey data. The incidence and duration of breast feeding are related to place of residence and it is more common and practised longer in rural than in urban areas. Many surveys have also found a correlation with age: among younger women it is less common and practised for a shorter time than among older women. Another factor with which lactation is related is education – women with higher levels of education practise it less frequently and for a shorter time than those with lower levels of education. Employment outside the home is also a significant factor. Several surveys have found that women who were employed and needed to return to their jobs soon after delivery, nurse less frequently and for a shorter time than those who are not working outside the home.

Consequences for infant mortality and morbidity

The change towards early weaning may not cause problems in well-to-do and middle-class families, but its impact is very significant for families living in poverty. There is ample evidence to show that replacement of breast feeding by bottle feeding at an early age in a poor socio-economic environment leads to an increased incidence of infant malnutrition, morbidity and mortality. In particular, the incidence of severe malnutrition during the first year rises as a result of 'weaning diarrhoea'. Cow's milk or infant formulas for bottle feeding are usually too expensive for a poor family to buy consistently for a number of months. Infant formulas, when properly used, take up an extremely large proportion of the household budget, and as a consequence mothers who find infant formulas too expensive may dilute the preparation or add rice water instead of cow's milk. Another problem is that formulas are prepared under unhygienic conditions leading to contamination.

Consequences for fertility

The decline in breast feeding not only has adverse consequences for infant morbidity and mortality but can raise fertility. As the duration of lactation falls, more and more women become exposed to the risk of pregnancy at earlier and earlier times after the last delivery. Where breast feeding becomes less common birth intervals become shorter, unless the use of contraception increases at the same time. An example of the impact of the decline of lactation on birth intervals is provided in Figure 3.

These data refer to birth intervals prior to the second birth of successive generations of North American Indian women living in the James Bay area in Canada. No modern contraception is practised there and it can clearly be seen that younger generations of mothers (those who had their second child when they were young at the time of the survey in 1968) had much shorter birth intervals than their older counterparts (those who were much older at the time of the survey in 1968 and who had their second child much earlier). It could be demonstrated that this shortening of birth intervals was to a large extent due to changes in lactation practices over a 20-year period, as Figure 3 indicates. Similar declines in birth intervals and consequent rises in fertility have been reported for other Indian and Eskimo groups living in Canada and Alaska. In another study concerning Canadian Eskimos, it was reported that the crude birth rate increased from 40 to 64 per 1000 in a period of 20 years, largely as a consequence of the introduction of bottle feeding. These changes in fertility, as a consequence of changes in lactation, could be easily monitored because these populations were rather isolated. In other countries, such changes are much more difficult to document because of the impact of many other factors in addition to lactation on birth intervals and fertility.

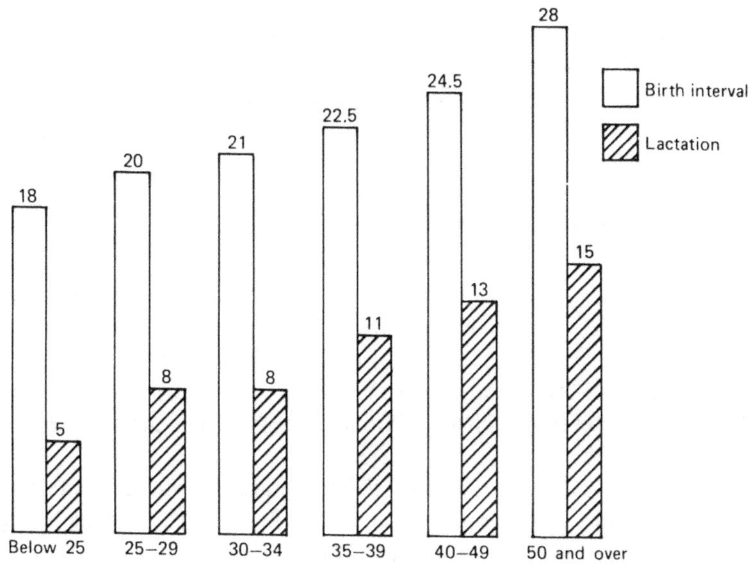

Figure 3 Relationship of lactating and birth intervals by age of mother, James Bay Indians, Canada. (Adapted from Romaniuk (1973) Tables 3 and 9)

Measures to protect breast feeding

It is, of course, easy to advocate continued use of breast feeding because of its advantages for mother and child, but it is quite another matter to indicate how to achieve this. Basic to all efforts to encourage breast feeding is the recognition that women should be able to fulfil a dual role – to bear and rear children as well as undertake activities outside the home. The situation for many urban women of developing countries is that if they choose to engage in activities outside the home, some activities related to child rearing will suffer and breast feeding is one of them. Faced with this dilemma, it is quite understandable that many choose to work outside the home and that breast feeding is consequently sacrificed.

The decline of breast feeding is inevitable as long as this conflict between the two roles of women continues to exist. Measures should, therefore, be taken to enable women to carry out their dual role inside and outside the house adequately. Such measures include legislation in favour of breast feeding (e.g. duration of maternity leave and job protection during such leave). Other legislative possibilities relate to attempting to correct the abuses of unethical advertising and promotion of infant formulas. Measures should also be taken concerning organization of health services (arrangements in maternity wards of hospitals and support for breast feeding in hospitals). Finally, health education should be initiated concerning the benefits and usefulness of breast feeding.

LACTATION AND MODERN CONTRACEPTION

There is a tendency to assume that contraceptive measures are unknown or are not practised in developing countries, because no modern contraceptive methods are used. In this chapter it has been demonstrated, however, that birth intervals from 30 to 36 months are achieved in many countries through prolonged breast feeding with or without support of abstinence from sexual relations after birth.

It is clear that prolonged breast feeding should be encouraged in many developing countries. This should be done in the first place to protect the health of children, because as we have seen, sharp decreases in lactation in poverty-stricken areas will lead to higher infant morbidity and mortality.

Lactation should also be advocated as a traditional birth-spacing method in areas where prolonged lactation is common. Introduction of modern contraceptives, in particular combined oral contraceptives, may even be counter-productive. A study in Manila, the Philippines, has found that the use-effectiveness of traditional methods can equal or exceed that of modern methods. Continuation of the use of oral contraceptives was similar to the duration of lactation amenorrhoea. In other words, women replaced a traditional practice by a modern method and nothing was gained in the process. Actually there was a loss if one takes into account increased risks to the health of the child.

In areas in developing countries where breast feeding is declining rapidly, family planning methods should be introduced to prevent birth intervals from decreasing and fertility from increasing. In other words, contraceptive methods should be adopted by these populations to compensate for declines in lactation amenorrhoea and/or postpartum abstinence.

Whenever modern contraceptives are introduced, it should be done taking into account the existence of traditional birth-spacing methods – that is emphasis should not only be on limiting family size but also on birth spacing. There are societies where birth spacing is acceptable to certain categories of the population whereas limiting family size is not yet acceptable. Emphasis on birth spacing alone will not solve the population problem which is emerging or existing in many countries, but in several societies it is the most acceptable way of introducing contraception. Contraception should also be introduced making use of the argument that such methods will not only be of assistance in achieving an adequate birth interval, but will enable women to breast feed for a reasonable amount of time.

Limitations of breast feeding as a birth-spacing method

In spite of the fact that lactation has been advocated here as a birth-spacing method in areas where it is well established (and where modern contraception methods are not likely to be widely available), its limitations should be realized.

* Variability in the resumption of menstruation is considerable. Although the average duration of amenorrhoea can be relatively long (an average of one year) – menstruation returns much earlier than this average for a considerable proportion of women. Breast feeding is definitely an effective spacing method for populations as a whole, but not for the proportion of women who resume menstruation early. For others menstruation will return later than average and if they adopt a contraceptive at the time normally advised they will involve themselves in a redundant effort.
* From 3–7% of women are likely to conceive during lactation amenorrhoea at the time of the first ovulation after birth which precedes the first menstrual period (if conception does not occur). Lactation, therefore, is by no means a perfect contraceptive method and women should initiate the use of contraception prior to the first ovulatory cycle after birth and not after return of the first menses. Unfortunately, a cheap, reliable and easy-to-use ovulation detection method is not available.
* In a healthy population the duration of lactation amenorrhoea may not last more than one year to 15 months at most. However, this provides considerable protection and, as we have seen, compares favourably with the use-effectiveness of oral contraceptives in a number of areas. There are, of course, other populations where the use-effectiveness of modern contraceptives in terms of length of use is much better than that achieved through lactation amenorrhoea.

* The nutritional requirements of the child must also be kept in mind. Full breast feeding should last until 4–6 months after birth and lactation as a supplementary source of nutrition should continue for 1–2 years after birth. A period of lactation amenorrhoea ranging beyond 12–15 months after birth corresponds, therefore, with periods of lactation which are not desirable from a nutritional point of view.

In view of these limitations, it is understandable that there are countries where breast feeding is practised together with postpartum abstinence. It may be that breast feeding alone is not considered sufficient to provide adequate protection against the risk of pregnancy.

Choice of contraceptive methods and time of introduction

The limited effectiveness of lactation raises the question as to which modern methods of contraception need to be adopted in the postpartum period and at what point in time after birth. As far as the choice of methods is concerned, the following conclusions can be drawn on the basis of research that has been carried out on this topic.

* Combined oral contraceptives containing oestrogen may have a negative effect on the amount of milk produced and may lead to early termination of lactation. In particular, pills with a high degree of oestrogen should not be used by lactating women and certainly not before six months postpartum. Low-dosage oestrogenic pills have much less effect on milk production and are more acceptable.
* There is no evidence of adverse effects of the IUD and other non-hormonal forms of contraception with respect to milk production and therefore such methods are preferred methods for postpartum women.
* Progestogenic and long-term injectable contraceptives have been shown to have no demonstrable effects on milk volume or composition. They are, however, not recommended methods, in particular during full lactation, because it is unknown whether some of the contents of these drugs are transferred via the milk to the infant and whether this has negative consequences for the infant.

A last issue to be considered is the most appropriate time to start with contraceptive methods in the postpartum period. There are various possibilities – contraception can be initiated immediately postpartum; at a certain point in time after birth, say 3 or 6 months; after changing from full to partial breast feeding; or after return of menstruation. The importance of several factors needs to be weighed.

From a pragmatic point of view, it is of course preferable to advise women who delivered in a hospital to start using contraception immediately postpartum since many of them will not return to the hospital soon after birth. However, other factors also need to be considered. In societies where breast feeding is prolonged, provision of contraceptives immediately postpartum will lead to a considerable period of overlap between lactation amenorrhoea and protection provided by modern contraception and in such societies this policy should probably not be followed.

CONCLUSIONS

Lactation is common in most developing societies and often lasts over one year. Breast feeding has a considerable impact on fertility in general and birth intervals in particular. Lactation achieves its birth-spacing effect by delaying the resumption of ovulation, but unfortunately there is no way of predicting when ovulation will return and wide variation exists between women, so that lactation has serious limitations as a contraceptive for the individual couple.

Lactation is declining in many developing countries, with adverse consequences for infant mortality as well as fertility. Modern contraception is sometimes little more than a substitute for traditional birth spacing due to breast feeding. Policies need to be established to protect traditional birth spacing methods. While it may be impossible to halt the trend away from breast feeding. Policies need to be established to protect traditional birth-introducing modern methods of contraception the existence of traditional methods should be taken into account.

Note: The information summarized in this chapter comes from various sources. These sources have not been quoted by the author, but can be found in the bibliography.

Bibliography

Crosignani, P. G. and Robyn, C. (eds.) (1977). *Prolactin and Human Reproduction.* (London: Academic Press)

Gray, R. H. (1975). Breastfeeding and Maternal and Child Health. *IPPF Medical Bulletin,* **9,** 61

Elliott, K. and Fitz Simmonds, D. W. (eds.) (1976). *Breast-feeding and the Mother,* CIBA Foundation Symposia 45 (Amsterdam: Excerpta Medica)

Jelliffe, D. and Jelliffe, P. (1977). *Human Milk in the Modern World.* (New York: Oxford University Press)

Mosley, W. H. (ed.) (1977). *Nutrition and Human Reproduction.* (New York: Plenum Press)

Parkes, A., Thomson, A., Potts, M. and Herbertson, M. (eds.) (1977). *Fertility Regulation during Human Lactation.* (Cambridge: Galton Foundation)

Rosa, F. (1975). Breast-Feeding in Family Planning. *P.A.G. Bulletin,* **5**, 5

Romaniuk, A. (1973). Modernization and natural fertility: the case of James Bay native Indians, in *Natural Fertility,* International Union for the Scientific Study of Population, Liège, Belgium

World Fertility Survey (1977, 1978). *Country Reports.*

SECTION TWO

Successful Family Planning Programmes

Successful family planning programmes are reviewed from a range of cultures: from Buddhist countries (Thailand and Sri Lanka), Islamic nations (Indonesia and Bangladesh) and from India and Japan. They involve different modalities of fertility regulation. In Japan, Sri Lanka and Bangladesh, contraceptives are sold at a price adjusted to the income of the consumer. In Thailand and Bali, the community is involved in the distribution of pills and condoms. All these schemes reach out to serve the needs of the poor and the very poor. Some programmes include referral for the surgical means of family planning. In Bombay, sterilization and abortion are offered in a busy clinic at a price many relatively poor people can afford and at a real cost which is lower than government institutions that offer the same procedures.

Successful programmes are united by three characteristics: they have strong, capable management, they emphasize the philosophy of marketing and try to meet the needs and perceptions of people as fully as possible and they are partially or totally self-sufficient in financial terms.

4

Using the local community – Bali, Indonesia

Ida Bagus Astawa

BACKGROUND 56

HISTORY OF THE BALI FAMILY PLANNING PROGRAMME AND ORGANIZATIONAL STRUCTURE 57

THE NATIONAL FAMILY PLANNING PROGRAMME 57

The National Family Planning Coordinating Board structure 58

THE BALI FAMILY PLANNING PROGRAMME 59

Motivation and education 59

Contraceptive services 59

Training 59

THE *BANJAR* SYSTEM 60

Why use the Banjar *system?* 61

How the Banjar *system is involved* 62

PRIVATE SECTOR 62

MENSTRUAL REGULATION 63

FERTILITY EFFECTS 63

WHY WAS THE PROGRAMME SUCCESSFUL? 65

Emphasis on promoting IUDs 68

Use of local social structure 69

CONCLUSIONS 69

BACKGROUND

Through a carefully designed and systematically implemented family planning programme, built on a traditional community organization, two-thirds of the eligible couples in Bali, Indonesia now use a modern method of contraception and the birth rate has fallen by 35% in 6 years (1970–76).

The island of Bali is one of the 27 provinces of the Republic of Indonesia. It occupies an area of 5711 square kilometres, or about 10 times the area of Singapore or three times the island of Oahu, Hawaii and is located immediately to the east of Java. With an estimated population (1977) of 2.3 million, the population density (about 400 persons per square kilometre) is high, especially for an almost entirely rural population. The majority of the population is Hindu, unlike the rest of Indonesia which is predominantly Moslem. The population of Indonesia in 1977 was about 141 million, making it the fifth most populous nation in the world. 47% of the total land area of Bali is cultivated; however, only 30% of the cultivated land (14% of the total land area) is suitable for growing rice, the staple of the Balinese diet.

Politically, the island is divided into eight regencies (*kabupaten*), the boundaries of which date back to the eight kingdoms that existed prior to the Dutch conquest of 1907. Each regency is divided into *kecamatan* (subdistricts) and each *kecamatan* is divided into villages. There are 50 *kecamatans* and 564 villages. Each village is further subdivided into *banjar* (community organization or hamlet) and there are 3727 *banjars* in the whole of Bali. It is the *banjar* organization which has been one of the keys to successful family planning in Bali. The average population of a village is 4000 people and a *banjar* consists of 50–100 households. There are no cities of notable size. The population of the largest city, Denpasar, is only about 100 000. Only 9.7% of the population were classified as urban in the 1971 census. Before the recent increases in Indonesia's oil revenues, Indonesia's per capita income was among the lowest in the world, estimated at US $80 in 1970. In 1973 the per capita income became US $150 and in 1974 became US $170 and in 1975 US $180.

The 1971 census revealed that educational attainment was low among Balinese women, 64.8% having no formal schooling, 18.1% less than six years, and with only 13.2% having completed the six-year elementary school programme. Less than 4% had progressed beyond elementary school. In 1971 73.3% of the economically active male population were farmers, 16.8% did manual work and 9.9% were in sales, clerical or higher status positions. Of the female population aged 15–44, only 31% were economically active and, of these, half were employed in agriculture. Thus in terms of urbanization, income, education and employment, Bali might appear rather ill-suited to the successful promotion of family planning.

The total fertility rate (TFR) in 1965–1970 was 5.8, the crude birth rate (CBR) 43.9 and the crude death rate was about 19 per thousand. Bali's recent high growth rate has left a young population with 43% below age 15. Migration has had a negligible role in population change according to the 1971 census. During the entire 1960s emigration exceeded immigration by only 5000, while during the three years immediately preceding the census immigration slightly exceeded emigration. Of a Balinese population of 2.1 million, as measured by the 1971 census, 460 306 (21.7%) were women aged 15–44, but because of the relatively late age of marriage only 306 846 were currently married. Therefore, in 1971 the number of couples eligible for family planning services (as indicated by the number of married women aged 15–44) constituted 14.5% of the total population.

HISTORY OF THE BALI FAMILY PLANNING PROGRAMME AND ORGANIZATIONAL STRUCTURE

The Indonesian Planned Parenthood Association (IPPA) was established in 1957 in Jakarta as a voluntary organization and is a member of the IPPF, London. However, the political situation at that time was unfavourable and the spread of the idea of family planning was very slow. The government, aware of the vast size of Indonesia (it is one of the eight largest countries in the world with an area of 1.9 million square kilometres), pursued a pronatalist policy. Nevertheless, motivation was done carefully and among selected people, beginning with the more educated and among medical and paramedical personnel.

In Bali the IPPA established a branch in 1961, but only simple methods were made available. The metal IUD was introduced for the first time in Bali in the late fifties by a West German gynaecologist who worked in the Department of Obstetrics of Sanglah Hospital, Denpasar. Only about 50 women accepted the method. In 1963 the IPPA introduced Lippe's loops in Sanglah Hospital as a pilot project. In the two years 1963–1965 there were 325 IUD insertions, the acceptors mostly consisting of paramedical personnel and village women around the capital.

THE NATIONAL FAMILY PLANNING PROGRAMME

In 1966 General Suharto was elected as the new president of the Republic of Indonesia and the political situation regarding family planning changed markedly. The IPPA held the first national congress in 1967, 10 years after its foundation. In its congress the IPPA recommended a national family planning programme, arguing that family planning was essential for the welfare of the people. The government response was positive, as proved by the first presidential speech in front of the parliament on August 16, 1967, where the role of family planning was emphasized for the welfare of the present and for the next generation.

In line with this policy, the government established a National Family Planning Institution, which was a semi-governmental body, using government facilities (clinics, doctors, paramedical personnel and the mobile information unit of the Department of Information). The government supported the family planning programme implemented by the IPPA. In 1970 the government reorganized the national management of the programme by establishing a National Family Planning Coordinating Board (NFPCB or BKKBN in Indonesian) and since this time the government has been fully responsible for the programme.

The objectives of the National Family Coordinating Board programme were to:

* make a 50% decrease in the fertility of Indonesian women by the year 2000 compared with fertility in 1970;
* recruit in the first 5 year plan, beginning in the fiscal year 1970–71, 6 million new acceptors with the goal of averting 1.7 million births;
* decrease in the same 5 years the growth rate of Indonesia by 0.8%.

The estimated annual growth rate of Indonesia in 1970 was 2.6 to 2.8%. In the first 5 year plan the family planning programme was concentrated on the six provinces of Java and Bali which are the most densely populated areas of Indonesia. In the second five year plan, beginning 1974, 10 additional provinces joined the programme. In the third five year plan, starting 1979 another 11 provinces will be brought into the programme which will then cover the whole nation (27 provinces).

The National Family Planning Coordinating Board structure

The National Family Planning Coordinating Board is a coordinating body to bring together family planning activities implemented by a number of governmental units:

* Department of Health, which is responsible for medical services;
* Department of Information, which is responsible for mass communication;
* Department of the Army, which is responsible for medical services in the armed services;

* Department of Education, responsible for population education and several private units (e.g. IPPA, Church Council and Muhammadiah).

THE BALI FAMILY PLANNING PROGRAMME

In line with the national family planning programme the Balinese programme consists of three components:

* Information, education and communication (IEC);
* Contraceptive services;
* Support components – training, financial, logistic and administrative.

Besides these three components, this discussion will emphasize the *banjar* system, where a traditional community organization has been used as a base for family planning activities. In addition to the national programme, the author will mention the private sector, especially the Dharma Dutta Foundation, which is sponsored by the Pathfinder Fund, and the sterilization programme, which is sponsored by the International Project of the Association for Voluntary Sterilization (IPAVS). A final important contribution to family planning in Bali has been the practice of menstrual regulation by some private medical practitioners.

Motivation and education

Since Bali is a mountainous island it is easier to recruit male field workers who can walk or ride a bicycle than female field workers. Field workers are recruited from the local village and are required to have completed at least junior high school and be a minimum of 18 years of age. The training of field workers is done in the Provincial Training Centre and goes on for 3 weeks (2 weeks theory and 1 week in the field).

Contraceptive services

The contraceptive services are provided by doctors in the 150 family planning clinics and 6 hospital post-partum programmes. In addition, there are 12 private clinics sponsored by the IPPA and the Dharma Dutta Foundation. However, as the number of doctors available for the work is limited, midwives have been trained to insert IUDs since 1972.

Training

Training plays a very important role in the programme. Bali has a provincial training centre which was established in 1968 with the sponsorship of the IPPA and all categories of training are carried out, including that of field workers, midwives, doctors, community leaders, religious leaders, artists (traditional drama players and shadow puppet players), leaders of women's organizations and school teachers.

Under the leadership of the chairman of the National Family Planning Coordinating Board of Bali, cooperation between this body and the director of the Provincial Training Centre is very good. The chairman of the National Family Planning Coordinating Board and his staff became guest lecturers for all categories of training, so that the two organizations speak one language in training the personnel needed for the programme. This is important since it would have been possible for the National Family Planning Coordinating Board to make a policy clarifying the mode of action of IUDs as preventing conception, but for the Provincial Training Centre to have taught a theory that said IUDs prevent nidation which could be interpreted as abortion. Of course, there are many other administrative and technical problems that have had to be clarified by the programme administration so there is no gap between the personnel who work in the field and the policy makers on the Provincial National Family Planning Coordinating Board.

THE *BANJAR* SYSTEM

A *banjar* is a traditional community organization at sub-village level. The origin of the system is unknown, but some old village leaders say that the *banjar* existed even before the Besakih Temple, the mother temple of Bali, which is located at the foot of Mount Agung, the highest mountain in Bali. If this is correct, then the *banjar* system is more than 1000 years old.

Banjars are made up of male heads of households. The average *banjar* contains 100 households and there are over 3500 *banjars* in Bali. Most *banjars* bind together a geographical unit, although some link a number of families or clans. In this latter case, a man in one village may then be a member of a *banjar* in another village. The *banjar* has a periodical meeting which is located in the *banjar* hall, a multipurpose building which acts as a place for preparing a temple ceremony, cock-fighting, practising the village orchestra (*gamelan*), traditional village dancing, performing entertainments and for preparing for cremation. Most *banjars* meet regularly (Table 1) and normally 100% of the membership attends because there is a system of *banjar* fines. Every absent member must pay Rp 100 (25 cents US) if he sent a message and he could not come and twice as much if he did not send a message. If a member is late by one hour he must pay Rp 50. Meetings are devoted to discussing the development of the community and religious affairs. Meetings are chaired by a leader *(kelian)* elected every 5 years.

TABLE 1 Frequency of *banjar* meetings

	Percentage
Monthly (Balinese month = 35 days)	71.3
Quarterly	3.3
Six-monthly	10.9
Other	14.5

Why use the *banjar* system?

A deliberate choice was made to build family planning around the *banjar* system for three purposes. Firstly, the *banjar* was used to institutionalize the small family norm within the community, using the *banjar* meeting as the medium. When the programme started in the early 1970s many women shied away from having an IUD insertion because they felt family planning was not an acceptable thing to do in the community. Such attitudes were changed by discussing family planning at the *banjar* meeting and showing it was good for people to adopt a method such as an IUD.

Secondly, the *banjar* system was to accumulate the statistics needed in planning and to record acceptors. In Indonesia there is a centralized reporting and recording system which is part of the National Family Planning Coordinating Board. This system is limited to monitoring the new acceptors and their characteristics. The data from each clinic is sent twice a month to Jakarta and processed on a computer. This system makes it possible to follow the cumulative total of new acceptors and, as the continuation rate for each method is known, it is possible to calculate the current use or prevalence rate. But by using the *banjar* system more accurate data is accumulated since current users are recorded each month.

Thirdly, the *banjar* system is used in a community-based service delivery system. One hundred and fifty clinics for the rural area of Bali are not enough for 564 villages and 3727 *banjars* scattered all over the island. By using the *banjar* system it is possible to link information and service about family planning and bring these two mutually related elements as close to the community as possible. The *kelian* can act as a depot holder for oral contraceptives, condoms and vaginal tablets.

How the *banjar* system is involved

Under the supervision and assistance of the National Family Planning Coordinating Board field workers, the *kelian* registers all eligible couples (*elco*) in the community and makes a map of each house with an *elco*. On the the map a different colour is used for IUD acceptors (blue), pill acceptors (red), condom acceptors (green) and a blank box is left for those who have not yet accepted a modern method. Each month the family planning situation in the village is reviewed, using the map. In order to do family planning work, the *kelian* is trained for three days in the Provincial Training Centre in Denpasar. The prevalence of contraceptive use in the island has risen every year and according to the *Banjar* Report of March 1978, 269 168 eligible couples, or 11.75% of the total number of the population (2 289 800), are now registered in the *banjar* system. Of this number 173 844 are using family planning – or 64.6% of all eligible couples. The IUD is the predominant method (Table 2).

TABLE 2 Contraceptive use (Bali, 1978)

Method	*Number*	*Percentage*
Pill	29 397	16.9
IUD	120070	69.1
Condoms	17 194	9.9
Spermicides	323	0.2
Tubectomy	5293	3.0
Vasectomy	1018	0.6
Injectable contraceptive	549	0.3

PRIVATE SECTOR

The private sector played an important role in initiating the work in Bali, in supplementing current activities and in exploring the addition of new methods to the programme. In 1967 the IPPA branch opened the first three family planning clinics in the island and in 1968 the Provincial Training Centre was established. As there are only one hundred and fifty clinics funded by the

National Family Planning Coordination Board, there are many isolated villages which are not covered by the national programme and the private sector still has an important role in service as well as in training.

In 1972 the Dharma Dutta Foundation in Bali sponsored by the Pathfinder Fund established twelve additional clinics. In 1974 the Dharma Dutta Foundation sponsored by the International Project of the Association for Voluntary Sterilization began offering sterilization services. Practically all the men and women obtaining sterilization since that time have been funded by IPAVS.

MENSTRUAL REGULATION

In December 1973 a doctor from Bali was invited to attend a first menstrual regulation conference in Honolulu, Hawaii (see also Chapter 10). A number of regulation kits were brought back and the doctor trained and supplied fourteen other interested physicians. The method has been and remains controversial. The public debate on menstrual regulation occurred in 1975 between doctors and involved even the public and newspapers. Since then only two doctors in Bali have continued practising menstrual regulation, but even so the number of cases is still increasing. The cumulative total of cases rose from 1000 in 1974, to 3000 in 1975, 6000 in 1976 and 9000 cases in 1977. In other words, there are now about 3000 menstrual regulation procedures a year and some commentators believe that the adoption of menstrual regulation by the people of Bali has had a powerful effect, strengthening the motivation for family planning.

FERTILITY EFFECTS

According to the data from the World Fertility Survey in 1976 the total fertility rate (TFR) in Bali was 3.8. As noted, between 1964–70 it had been 5.8 and it was calculated to have been 4.6 in 1974. Therefore the overall decline in fertility in the 6 years 1970–76 was 34.5% (Tables 3 and 4). Procedures have been devised for estimating couple-years of protection. In the fiscal year 1973–74 the programme directly provided 68 500 couple-years of protection and, as a result, 21.3% of potential couple-years of exposure to the possibility of conception were effectively protected by programme methods. Assuming the fertility 9 months later was correspondingly reduced, the programme was responsible for a decline in the birth rate of about 8 per 1000 during the calendar year 1974, or an estimated 21 000 births averted. If the programme were the only factor affecting fertility, the estimated crude birth rate would have declined from 43.9 around 1970 to 40.4 in 1972, to 37.7 in 1973 to 34.5 in 1974. In fact, the fall in the birth rate was even more rapid and the National Family Planning Coordinating Board estimated the crude birth rate as 28.0 in 1976.

TABLE 3 Estimated total fertility rate (TFR) Java–Bali provinces in 1976 and estimated percentage of fertility reduction since 1967–1970

Province	*Estimated TFR 1967–1970*	*Estimated TFR 1976*	*Reduction since 1967–1970*
Jakarta	5.12	4.5	11.8%
West Java	5.87	5.3	10.2%
Central Java	5.27	4.4	17.0%
Yogyakarta	4.69	4.4	6.4%
East Java	4.65	3.9	17.0%
Bali	5.83	3.8	34.5%

TABLE 4 Estimated fertility effects attributable to the programme, calendar years 1972–1974

Fertility	*1972*	*1973*	*1974*
Couple-years of protection during fiscal year (5 months before)	29 100	52 200	79 000
Couple-years of effective protection	24 200	44 200	68 500
Percentage reduction in fertility from 1965–1970 level	7.9	14.1	21.3
Number of births averted	7400	13 600	21 100
Estimated CBR* (allowing for estimated programme effects but not for non-programme effects)	40.4	37.7	34.5
Estimated TFR** (allowing for programme effects)	5.4	5.1	4.6

*CBR = Crude birth rate
**TFR = Total fertility rate

WHY WAS THE PROGRAMME SUCCESSFUL?

At first glance, Bali seems an inauspicious place to mount a successful family planning programme. Many factors would seem to encourage traditional high levels of fertility:

* per capita income is low;
* female educational attainment and labour force participation are low;
* industrial and commercial development are low;
* the people are noted for their devotion to religious practices and the arts rather than to more worldly concerns;
* the Balinese constitute a religious and ethnic minority in Indonesia, whereas the family planning programme is part of a national Indonesian policy rather than an indigenous development;
* there was little evidence of much practice of contraception before the programme;
* even since the programme has been in operation the ideal family size has remained close to four children; in the 1973 Fertility/Mortality Survey it was 3.8;
* childlessness is viewed as an affliction;
* traditional Balinese law excludes daughters from inheritance, thereby placing pressure on couples to have at least one surviving son. (Couples without natural sons, however, can obtain surrogates through marriage or adoption).

In addition, the programme encountered a number of administrative and operational problems:

* national level policies (such as the exclusion of sterilization procedures from the programme) are probably unnecessary in Bali but nevertheless are applied, limiting this method to private, non-governmental initiatives;
* the national administrative structure and procedures have been reorganized frequently with some initially disruptive effects;
* transport facilities are inadequate for the needs of supervisors and field workers;
* the recruitment of qualified personnel has suffered from the programme's inability to pay competitive salaries and to provide long-term job security, owing to the peculiar status of the National Family Planning Coordinating Board among government agencies;
* funds for programme activities or for payments that require special approval are sometimes months late in arriving at the provincial office;
* the joint effect of low salaries and late payment of referral fees has created a high rate of turnover among field workers.

Despite all these obstacles and problems the programme has been able to operate with demonstrable efficiency. The success of the programme indicates that the factors facilitating its operation are numerous and important enough to outweigh the impeding factors by a wide margin. The factors believed by the author to contribute most to programme success are discussed below under three headings: cultural, situational and programme factors.

When family planning began, there was concern about the possibility of resistance from the Hindu Bali religion. It was feared that some beliefs would prove at variance with the small family norm:

* in the Balinese pattern of belief every baby born brings its own benefit from heaven;
* the Balinese believe in reincarnation, so it might be thought that using an artificial method to prevent a birth might prevent a reincarnation.

Fortunately, the Balinese religion proved tolerant of family planning. There was good participation from religious leaders who developed the theme of small families using the story of *Panca Pandawa* (the five brothers). In this religious tale the five brothers of *Pandawa* consist of three single born children and a pair of twins and they attack and overcome the one hundred *Kurawa* brothers. The story was interpreted by religious leaders to mean quality (the five *Pandawa* brothers) is better than quantity (the one hundred *Kurawa* brothers).

A cultural tradition that has proved very useful to programme administrators in promoting a reduced family size is the method of *naming children*. A Balinese child is usually given a name consisting of three or four parts, an optional marker indicating sex and a name identifying the given name by which the person will be formally addressed. It is the birth order name that is of particular interest here. The most common names for the first four births in a family are as follows:

First born: *Wayan, Gde, Putu* (literally 'the oldest')
Second : *Made, Nengah* ('middle')
Third : *Nyoman* ('youngest')
Fourth : *Ketut* ('extra')

For fifth and later children, either the cycle is repeated or each child is named *Ketut*. Clearly, the system of naming supports a traditional ideal family size of three or four. In one survey of Balinese women in 1973 the most commonly mentioned ideal family size (four children) was attributed to this naming system. The family planning information and motivation programme personnel in Bali have been able to use the naming system as a justification for the provincial programme's official message that couples should limit their child-bearing to three children. The 1973 Fertility/Mortality Survey found that a majority (55.6 per cent) of Balinese women who already had three living children said that they did not want any more. The exact balance between the numerary system and the programme's emphasis on stopping at three, however, is not clear.

The Balinese pattern of land tenure is supportive of family limitation. Although on per capita basis the Balinese, especially in rural communities, are poor even in comparison with other developing areas, they are nevertheless able to realize the full benefits derived from their work rather than sharing their produce with non-productive land owners; share cropping and tenancy are rare in Bali. In keeping with the Balinese traditional cohesive social organization, much of the agricultural land is communally owned and operated, but the proceeds benefit the local community as a whole rather than enriching only a few persons.

According to the Fertility/Mortality Survey, of eligible women in cases where the husband is a farmer, fully 76% are self-employed and 10% are family workers, while only 14% work as agricultural labourers. As a result, farm families are probably more likely to feel that they have some control over their own welfare and therefore to be more receptive to family planning than would occur if they were being economically exploited by a few wealthy land owners.

In contrast to the rest of Indonesia, and to most of the developing world, traditional birth attendants (*dukun*) in Bali are male. As a result, Balinese women tend to be less inhibited about pelvic examinations or IUD insertions carried out by male physicians than in many other traditional societies. This factor was of critical importance in establishing the IUD as the main programme method, since almost all IUD insertions had to be performed by male physicians. Today, it is of less significance as most IUD insertions are now made by trained female midwives.

Not only are births in Bali traditionally attended by male midwives, but in rural areas a husband also often helps his wife during the delivery which, in turn, is usually witnessed by all the relatives of the family. Such openness about reproductive functions must greatly simplify the work of providing information about contraceptive methods, for example, persuading potential clients to undergo pelvic examinations and IUD insertion.

Among the programme factors leading to success has been a determination not to stop pushing forward when any particular level of success was achieved. Both information and motivation and clinical activities were involved in the 'extra drive' introduced in December 1972 when eight new vehicles were made available to the programme, one for each regency. These vehicles were used by mobile teams to take information and motivation activities and clinic services to villages. The extra drive relied principally on two-day visits by the mobile teams to outlying villages, preceded by preparatory activities carried out by the regular field workers in the area. The first day consisted of information and motivation activities with lectures, group discussions, testimonials by satisfied users, and movies in the evening. On the second day the clinic team went into action providing contraceptives (mostly IUDs).

Like most other family planning programmes, Bali's programme emphasizes efforts to provide information and motivation through home visits, posters, mobile film projection units and radio programmes. In addition, special family planning training courses have been conducted for professional actors in traditional theatre productions and for the men (*dalang*) who both narrate and manipulate the puppets in shadow plays. The objective of these courses was to encourage the performers to include family planning themes and messages in their highly popular productions (which always include much topical ad-libbing and joking in addition to the traditional stories). This integration of family planning information and motivation efforts in traditional media is thought to be at least as effective as the use of modern media, since the traditional media are widely seen and greatly appreciated on Bali.

The problem of providing clinical services to women who live far from the clinic is solved by taking the services to them. In Bali the scarcity of doctors is offset by the use of midwives for IUD insertion and pill prescription. Midwives make regular rounds outside the clinics, and often the house of the hamlet chief *(kelian banjar)* is used for IUD insertion in the field. Pill users are given three cycles at a time so that they do not need to return so often, thus making the method more attractive for the client and freeing the clinic personnel for other activities. Resupplies are kept by the *banjar* leader.

Emphasis on promoting IUDs

Unlike practically every other rural family planning effort in the world, the Balinese programme relies heavily on IUDs (Table 2). The majority of acceptors, therefore, select a method with an extremely high continuation rate. This preference is principally the result of a concerted effort by the programme administrators to promote the IUD combined with efforts to bring services close to the people. Field workers are trained to devote special attention to the IUD in providing information about the programme. Clinical personnel are interested in recommending IUDs above other methods, promote continuation among IUD users who are considering having the IUD removed or changing methods and encouraging users of other methods to shift to the IUD. The IUD is said to be more practical for hard-working village women since they need not worry about remembering to take pills every night or face the difficulty of finding a condom in the darkness of a village without electricity every time they have sex. It is important to prevent the spread of rumours such as 'the IUD can enter the stomach and give stomach pains' or 'the IUD can stick to the eye or head of the baby if an acceptor gets pregnant'. The programme administrator reacts rapidly to counter rumours through the family planning field workers.

The emphasis on the IUD is apparent not only in the proportion of acceptors who select the IUD and the large proportions who shift from the other methods to the IUD, but also in their knowledge of specific methods. Whereas in other provinces in Indonesia the pill is more widely known than the IUD, in Bali the reverse is true. According to the Fertility/Mortality survey, fully 68% of the respondents named the IUD without prompting when asked what methods they had heard of. By contrast, only 40% named the pill without prompting, 8% named the condom and still fewer named other methods.

Use of local social structure

A major part of the programme's strength is drawn from the cooperation received from local leaders and social organizations within the community. Much of the credit for this cooperation belongs to the Governor of Bali and regency chiefs (*bupati*) who urge local leaders to provide assistance to the family planning programme. Local leaders assist by integrating family planning into community meetings, by setting an example of practising family planning themselves and by encouraging community residents in need of family planning to join the programme.

In addition, every community in Indonesia has a branch of the national women's organization (the Family Welfare Association) which places special emphasis on upgrading the role of women in development through training in literacy, home economics, cottage industry and the like. In recent years the promotion of family planning has been integrated into the objectives of the Family Welfare Association and its meetings are routinely used for dissemination of family planning information. In the light of the cohesiveness of communities in Bali such support is important to the success of the programme.

CONCLUSIONS

Despite a number of factors which could well have discouraged successful family planning in Bali, those aspects of the culture likely to encourage smaller families were sought out and maximized. Existing social structures were used as the foundation for service referrals and, when appropriate, for services themselves and even as a basis for monitoring the programme. While respecting ancient traditions and responding to the needs of the people a policy decision was made, and successfully implemented, to promote IUDs as the major method. Surgical methods are becoming more important but still depend on non-governmental organizations.

Bibliography

Hull, T. H., Hull, V. J. and Singarimbun, Masri (1977). Indonesia's family planning story: success and challenge. *Population Bulletin,* **32** (6), 1

Soetedjo Moeljodihardo and Pasons, J. S. (1977). Trends in achievements in the Indonesian family planning program. Paper presented at International Union for the Scientific Study of Population Seminar, Liège

Sujono, Harjono, S., Hartai Pandi, Astawa, Ida Bagus, Moeljono and Reese, T. H. (1976). *Village Family Planning – The Indonesian Model: Institutionalizing Contraceptive practice.* Technical Reports Series Monograph **13** (Jakarta: BKKBN)

Sujono, Harjono (1974). *The Adoption of an Innovation in a Developing Country.* Community and Family Study Center, University of Chicago

5

Involving the community – Thailand

Mechai Viravaidya
and
Malcolm Potts

INTRODUCTION 72
THAILAND 73
STRUCTURE AND MANAGEMENT 74
Genesis 74
Donor assistance 75
Objectives 76
PROGRAMME DESCRIPTION 76
Commodities 77
The village distributor 77
Supervision 78
THE CONSUMERS 79
The joy of family planning 79
ACHIEVEMENTS 82
Contraceptive use 82
Demographic 82
Towards self-sufficiency 84
Administration 88
PROBLEMS AND OPPORTUNITIES 88
Sterilization and abortion 89
Integrated projects 89
CONCLUSIONS 90

INTRODUCTION

Recent experience in Thailand has shown that it is possible to develop cost-effective, replicable, rural family planning services using the human resources to be found in any Third World village (Table 1). Such community-based family planning services can provide realistic levels of medical supervision, are culturally acceptable and come to be used by a significant proportion of fertile women within a short time. In the Thai case they have produced a measurable fertility decline within 2 years.

By the early 1970s the first generation of clinic-based family planning programmes were coming under critical review and a number of innovations were developing with greater potential to serve large numbers of users. It was appreciated that, while oral contraceptives have a measurable risk, particularly in western women, the hazards are more than offset by those of unplanned pregnancy. It came to be understood that a variety of personnel could responsibly distribute these compounds using the history of past illness and age of a potential user as a most important screening procedure.

In 1973 the Central Medical Committee of the International Planned Parenthood Federation (IPPF) concluded that whoever 'normally meets the health needs of the community, whether doctor, nurse, traditional practitioner, a pharmacist or storekeeper, can be an appropriate person to distribute oral contraceptives'. This policy received practical confirmation in various parts of the world, including Colombia, Brazil and Thailand itself. The first two experiments involved IPPF affiliates, the last a decision by the Thai Ministry of Health to permit trained midwives, as well as medical practitioners, to dispense the Pill in 1970. Oral contraceptive use rose from 8000 to 31 000 women inside one year.

As the narrow perspective of clinic-based family planning broadened, so other changes also took place. Social marketing schemes, in which the distribution of contraceptives was subsidized to levels appropriate to the disposable income of a community, were pioneered by Population Services International in Kenya and subsequently in Sri Lanka (Chapter 8). The significance of the condom as a method of family planning became more widely appreciated. In the case of oral contraceptives, trained community personnel who distributed Pills were compensated for their work by keeping a proportion of the selling price. The village distribution scheme in Colombia under Tomayo and Echeveria pioneered this approach. These ideas were brought together under a major policy decision of the IPPF Management and Planning Committee to create a special department for Community-Based Distribution (CBD) with its own budget for 1974 onwards.

The following chapter describes the planning, implementation, achievements and problems facing the CBD programme which the IPPF assisted in launching in Thailand in 1973/4. It provides a critical analysis of experience up until 1978 in the belief that it is an important model from which a great deal can be learnt. It pays particular attention to administrative and financial implications of the programme, as well as dealing with the structural elements and technical problems concerned.

The phrase 'community-based distribution' was coined by Malcolm Potts during the course of a meeting in Rio, Brazil. The words 'commercial distribution' were an inaccurate description of the kind of work that had grown up in Colombia and were offensive to many people working in voluntary family planning. The words 'non-clinical distribution', which were also used to describe early programmes, proved embarrassing to the medical profession and were also inaccurate as the emerging oral contraceptive distribution programmes in reality were a system of *delegated* medical supervision.

THAILAND

At the end of the Second World War Thailand had a population of 17.5 million; today there are 44 million people and an annual growth rate of 2.5%. The per capita income is $378 which is above the Asian average and the country remains a major rice exporter. But if progress is to continue, the rate of population growth must slow (45% of the population is below age 15). For example poverty and pressure of numbers ensure that although many Thai children enter primary education, 85% reach a maximum 4th grade. In 1976 over one million of the 19 million labour force were unemployed and even more were underemployed. Some of the rural health problems in Thailand are summarized in Table 1.

Thailand is a predominantly Buddhist country, but 5% of the population is Moslem. It has a constitutional monarchy and literally translated the name means 'land of the free'. Alone among its neighbours, Thailand was never colonized. Until 1956 the government paid bonuses to large families, but in 1964 the Ministry of Public Health began small-scale participation in family planning and in 1970 the Thai Cabinet acted on a policy statement from the National Economic Development Board to declare an official population policy. In 1976 national contributions to family planning were $2.9 million and the United Nations Fund for Population Activities, the United States Agency for International Development, the World Bank and the IPPF gave external assistance.

Community-Based Family Planning Services (CBFPS) experience is part of a national response to population and family planning problems which cuts across all social groups. It is one element in the step from policies and pilot

TABLE 1 Some rural health problems in Thailand

Ratio doctors : village patients	1:110 000
Thai doctors working outside Bangkok	33%
Rural children who are anaemic	90%
Home deliveries (1972)	87.7%
– attended by granny midwife	63.7%
– women receiving antenatal care	35.0%
Villages with health centres (1969)	8.7%
– time spent by auxiliary midwives waiting at clinic	26.2%
– time spent by auxiliary midwives delivering babies	0.2%

After Somsak and Debhanom (1977)

projects to meaningful national involvement which so many nations must take, but which to date few have achieved.

STRUCTURE AND MANAGEMENT

Genesis

Between July and November 1973 the first author began experimenting with a number of new ideas in the work of the Planned Parenthood Association of Thailand (PPAT). Encouraging results were obtained whenever indigenous personnel, whether village leaders, *molams* (itinerant entertainers), or other selected individuals were recruited to help with family planning. The community as a whole appeared to be responsive to improved availability of services. These small-scale efforts were assisted by the transfer of a grant for about $1000 from the first Hugh Moore Award which had gone to the new director of the IPPF's CBD Department. Slightly later, the Secretary General of the IPPF approved the transfer of $10000 to allow further testing of ideas. This quick and flexible response was an important element in establishing the programme and creating trust between the donor agency and those working in the field.

By the end of 1973, it was possible to plan a programme to explore the possibility of building an alternative non-clinic system of contraceptive distribution and promotion in rural areas. It became apparent that the idea was important, but, at the same time, insufficiently tested to make it an appropriate routine programme to be conducted by PPAT. Therefore, a separate entity (Community-Based Family Planning Services – CBFPS) was devised, allowing the required managerial flexibility and also insulating the important routine work of PPAT from any possibility of backlash in case of failure. A private, not-for-profit organization was set up and outline plans to implement a trial project in one district of 70 000 people won approval from the Ministry of Public Health of the Royal Thai Government. An advisory committee of Thai leaders and experts was created, including physicians, bankers and specialists in rural development.

Donor assistance

Pioneers in community-based distribution of contraceptives from around the world had been brought together as advisors to the IPPF on implementing and supporting the new programmes. The majority recommended launching an independent technical and financial assistance organization to encourage CBD projects. But the enthusiasts closest to the problem had to compromise in order to obtain sufficient resources and the new department grew in the womb of the IPPF, instead of cutting the umbilical cord.

In Thailand, unlike many other programmes (at least outside the Peoples' Republic of China), the planning and execution of the work was conducted without any significant input from western professional personnel. The donor staff thought it was their responsibility to discover and understand the nature of the ideas put forward, explain the needs and constraints of the IPPF, seek budget and commodity support and share in monitoring the evaluation of the programme in the hope that, if successful, it would pull additional resources into the IPPF network and could serve as a model for creating similar programmes in other countries. On this basis, colleagues working on opposite sides of the world, but united in a strong bond of trust and mutual respect, launched the programme in 1974.

In addition to the provision of resources, the IPPF donor relationship permitted the rapid transfer of ideas in and out of Thailand; for example, some sales ideas came from Europe. The authority of the IPPF Central Medical Committee helped counter local hesitancy about methods of pill distribution. In the opposite direction the impact of the Thai CBD programme was rapidly transmitted around the world in IPPF publications and through the wider media, being reported in the USA, Japanese and British newspapers, Asian magazines, *Reader's Digest* and on German and Swiss television.

Objectives

The primary objective was to test the possibility of using existing local personnel and channels of distribution to markedly expand access to and information about contraceptive methods and create new and increased demand for family planning beyond the level then reached by existing commercial and institutional endeavours. The underlying hypothesis was that careful identification, selection, training, motivation and supervision of community personnel and resources, together with the availability of contraceptives within these communities, would lead to an increase in the number of couples practising family planning and a consequent decline in fertility. It was anticipated that the greater geographical convenience of information, consultation and the availability of contraceptives, as well as the cultural acceptability of seeking and receiving advice from a resident member of one's own community would result in a higher demand and practice rate in rural communities. It has been found, for example, that the cost of time spent on travelling by rural couples to acquire contraceptive supplies was often greater than the cost of the supplies themselves. It was also noted that, although the primary health services of rural Thailand were improving, the great majority of primary health centres remained unstaffed by a qualified physician and that doctors in Thailand, as in all developing countries, were mainly concentrated in Bangkok and the provincial capitals; the ratio of doctors to patients often exceeding 1 to 100 000 in rural areas.

PROGRAMME DESCRIPTION

All the activities of the programme were carried out with the approval and close cooperation of the Royal Thai Government and all the achievements of the programme are attributed to the national family planning programme. CBFPS has three arms. The village programme will be described below. A public institution programme was set up to assist existing government and industrial organizations with a large membership and some medical infrastructure. In particular, the Teachers' Council Medical Centre provided an acceptable and accepting outlet for contraceptive supplies. Thirdly, a private sector programme was established to cover opportunities falling outside the first two programmes.

Commodities

The IPPF provided 'Blue Lady' (Norinyl) Pills through the generosity of USAID and bulk-purchased Eugynon from Schering, Germany. These were then resold at subsidized prices in the villages for approximately one third to one half of the commercial market price current in Thailand. In the case of Norinyl, the villager pays 5Bt ($0.25) and 9Bt ($0.45) for Eugynon. The distributor keeps 20% of the selling prices.

In October 1976 the Thai government reversed its earlier policy of charging for contraceptives and provided a free supply of oral contraceptives to anyone requesting it. Nationally, this led to an increase in total acceptors, but it caused a loss of income to health centres and posed a confusing problem for CBFPS acceptors: they could either put themselves out and get a free supply from the geographically limited government services or remain faithful to their village distributors. Some did change and in certain areas the previously rising graph of CBFPS acceptors plateaued off. A recent official evaluation concluded that the National Family Planning Board 'should reconsider its pricing policy'.

Interestingly, the ratio of 25 cent Pills to 45 cent Pills in the CBFPS programme has shifted from 1:7 in 1976 to 1:2.3 in 1977, showing that village consumers will pay for what they perceive to be an advantageous service, even in the presence of free distribution.

The village distributor

The backbone of the programme is the village distributor. Someone from each village is selected and trained to be a motivator and distributor of contraceptives. An effort has been made to recruit one distributor for every 500 to 1000 of population and by May 1978, 12 000 distributors had been trained from 150 districts covering a population of 15 million and 33% of all the villages in Thailand. Distributors receive one day's initial training and the opportunity of retraining at a later date. They are given a certificate which they are proud to display in their homes and those with the best records are rewarded by being invited to meetings in Bangkok. A continuous planned effort is made to promote their status within a community.

The distributors hold supplies of Pills and condoms; the point of distribution is identified by a large painted metal sign comparable to those used by soft drink manufacturers in the villages of the developing world. A simple record system has been devised, with each user allotted one line and looking more like a school register than the cumbersome record cards and folders still used in most family planning clinics. Distributors have found no difficulty in keeping the records required of them, but it is important to note that distributors are recruited for their personality and commitment and not according to any arbitrary criteria. For example, a small number of distributors are illiterate and use some other family member to complete the forms.

A stratified random sample of 450 distributors (about one fifth of the then total) was conducted in 1975. Just under two thirds of the distributors were male and three quarters of the male distributors were over 35, while the majority of female distributors were slightly younger. All but 1% of distributors had a full time occupation or profession (38% rice farmers; 39% shopkeepers; 7% crop farmers; 3% teachers). Among the other groups were postmen, village headmen, silk weavers, traditional midwives and traditional medicine men. Seventy one per cent of distributors also had a secondary occupation and, on the whole, they belong to an intelligent, ambitious, entrepreneurial group within society.

The distributors' only financial reward comes from the sale of contraceptives, but many have gained in respect from the rest of the community and it is encouraging on an individual basis to note the improvements which many of the distributors have made to their homes or shops during the course of their work.

Supervision

Distributors have two sources of supervision and advice. A local doctor is always involved in the programme, often participates in training and is known by the distributors as a source of help if they encounter any medical problems. The doctor receives a small payment for this part-time work. In addition a field supervisor is appointed as a full-time staff person in each district of population, ranging from 40 000 to 130 000. He or she supervises the work of distributors, delivers supplies and assists in the management of record-keeping and the follow-up of contraceptives users. Supervisors cover about 1000 sq. kilometres and travel by motor cycle (or by boat in some areas). They are responsible to a field officer stationed in Bangkok (or in the case of Northern Thailand, in Chiang Rai).

THE CONSUMERS

CBFPS extends into all regions of Thailand. Seventy per cent of the population assisted are farmers, 10–14% labourers and fewer than 5% business people or government employees. Over 70% of consumers own their own land and nearly all live in detached houses constructed from local materials. The average household has 5–6 members. In two thirds of cases there is only one bedroom.

Thailand has enjoyed political stability for a long time. It is a Third World country where the term developing is a meaningful one. Relatively short term changes and improvements are taking place in the life of the people. Most are very poor by western standards, but enjoy reasonable nutrition and a dignified way of life. Nevertheless, they are vulnerable to crop failures and can easily fall into the hands of money lenders. From the point of view of material possessions in the regions covered by the programme, 80% had a radio, over a quarter a bicycle, and 1 in 10 a sewing machine. One in 50 had some sort of motor vehicle and 7.3% a motor cycle. However, 40% of farmers still used draught animals for ploughing.

Only 10–16% of the women and 6% of the husbands had no school education whatsoever, but less than 5% of the women completed more than 4 years of primary education. Marriage is almost universal in Thai villages and remarriage relatively common amongst older women. Only 3% of married women between the ages of 15 and 44 had never been pregnant. One third had one to two children, over a quarter three to four and one fifth reported seven pregnancies or more. Among women over 35 only one fifth had three children or less and among women over 40, 80% had four or more children and 65% had seven or more children.

As in a great many contemporary developing countries, there was a big gap between ideal and achieved family size. Only 7% of women in the project areas thought that seven or more children was an ideal family size. About 97% of women already had some knowledge of family planning and 91% approved of family planning in theory. However, in rural areas a good deal of suspicion of oral contraceptives remains and nearly 40% of married women felt that birth control pills are harmful to a woman's health. By the time the project was launched the bulk of village women felt that contraceptives should only be prescribed by a doctor.

The joy of family planning

Sex and humour should never be too far apart. Yet, most family planning programmes approach the topic of contraception in a joyless, anaemic way. In the CBFPS programme a consistent, bold, imaginative policy has been followed, using the amusing side of contraception to sustain interest and the funny side of life as a way into the serious aspects of family planning and population.

The condom has become a symbol of the programme as well as part of services. For example, it is common practice at large meetings to invite a group of men from the audience to compete in a condom race. Each is given a condom to unwrap, blow up and burst. No one in the audience can maintain a pompous attitude towards contraceptives handled in such a public way; neither can they feel that they are dirty, undercover things. By humour and by trivializing the actual mechanics of contraception so that it is no longer frightening, the attitudes of individuals and ultimately the attitudes of the nation are being changed.

The need for contraception knows no barriers of language, social class or political attitude. In 1975 the Royal Thai Government was having top level meetings with representatives of the newly unified nation of Vietnam. It has always been the policy of the CBFPS workers to carry condoms for distribution, even out of working hours. The opportunity arose, at an evening reception, for the CBFPS director to meet the Vietnamese deputy foreign minister and to the astonishment of the gathering, the fraternal greetings of one section of the Thai people were symbolically presented to the Vietnamese delegation by packets of condoms.

Next day, the Thai press commented on the episode, some in good humour, but others condemned it. The programme and the Director were said in some quarters to have 'gone too far this time'. However, a few days later the North Vietnamese representative asked to be able to receive members of CBFPS. It was acknowledged that the original episode was a gimmick, but it turned out to be a successful one and the subsequent discussions were useful and marked by a desire on both sides to learn from the other's experience of family planning and population.

Everything that is sold for fund raising has a family planning message. Even socks contain a pair of condoms and CBFPS panties are 'guaranteed not to cause pregnancy!' 'Proud Pete', the little anthropomorphic penis that puts on a condom, rises up in various places from T-shirts to contraceptive packaging. Various slogans, such as an adaptation of the Buddhist saying 'many children make you poor' are also used. The emphasis is on the everyday nature of family planning.

Children have come to play a key role. Tens of thousands can now sing a family planning song, based on a traditional children's rhyme. It describes the sadness of too many children who often have not enough to eat – but ends on a happy note: the distributor will tell your parents where to get the Pill, IUD or sterilization. Six-year-olds know if their mummies use the Pill and may even collect it. In Thailand, something a child handles becomes innocent and clean.

The overall approach comes together in a single sheet foldover leaflet

CBFPS workers carry. On the front the scriptural quotation 'many children make you poor' validates and identifies the programme, inside one coloured condom in a transparent envelope amuses and provides a practical introduction to contraception (with Proud Pete showing anyone unfamiliar with the method how to use it). A postal reorder form is available and on the back

> *If we allow the present birth rate to continue unchecked over the next 30 years, and even with double cropping of rice, there will not be enough rice to feed our population. Our present export of rice will sadly become an import. Today, the population is increasing at 2.5% per year: each minute three births occur while only one person dies, leaving an increase of two people every minute.*
>
> *While it is widely recognized that the endeavours of the* Ministry of Public Health *and the* Community-Based Family Planning Services *are considerable, resulting in a reduction of the population growth rate from 3.1% to 2.5% over the last five years, it is not enough. We must reduce our growth rate over the next five years to 2.1%.*
>
> *Each family should only have two or three children. Medical science and commonsense tells us clearly that the shorter the gap between births, the greater is the risk to both mother and child. We should therefore allow a space of four years between each child.*
>
> *May I leave this sincere request for my beloved and respected countrymen to practise family planning.*
>
> *Thanin Kraivichien*
> *Prime Minister of Thailand*
> *October 1977*

the demographic problems of Thailand are summarized in one table – and from rice farmer to demographer, the fact of two extra persons a minute is equally memorable. The Prime Minister has been photographed holding up such a leaflet and the hostesses from the red light areas of Bangkok know all about them.

ACHIEVEMENTS

Contraceptive use

The programme has had a local, national and international effect. It has provided a needed and acceptable local service. By the end of 1978 a cumulative total of 231 000 Pill users had entered the village programme. The village programme is monitored from the distributor record forms and by annual household impact and customer surveys. The goal of the programme has always been to promote family planning, not to propagate a single method of fertility control, and while oral contraception has been the central and most visible aspect of the programme, the common obsession with continuation rates has been replaced by a broader classification of family planning use. In addition, to gain a fuller insight, distributor records have been cross referenced with annual sample household impact and consumer surveys. Thirty to forty per cent of consumers were trial users of oral contraceptives who experimented with the method as one fertility regulation option. An equal number became acceptors who chose this as their definitive method, others dropped out (approximately 5%) or had used the Pill previously and were returned acceptors (approximately 1%); 10–16% were intermediate users or difficult to classify.

Demographic

Whereas many programmes shy away from any measure of demographic change, CBFPS made measurement of total fertility change a priority. The sample question 'are you pregnant or do you think you are pregnant?' was asked of married women aged 15–44 years in the sample surveys before the programme was initiated and after it had been running for 2 years (Table 2). Fertility is declining throughout Thailand, but fell most rapidly in those villages with CBFPS distribution. In areas covered by the programme women claimed that between 65% of pregnancies (South) and 85% (North) had been planned, the ideal number of children fell from 4 to 3 and contraceptive practice jumped from 10 to 60%. Approval of family planning, confidence in sterilization and other measures of acceptance and knowledge also improved. Seventy two per cent of consumers spent less than 15 minutes travelling to obtain contraceptives; 17% 15–25 minutes and only 6% more than half an hour.

Negative responses to the programme were few. Only 0.9% did not have sufficient faith in the ability of the distributor, and 2.3% commented that they did not like the programme because there was no physical examination.

TABLE 2 Fertility decline with Community-Based Family Planning Services (CBFPS)

Region	*Areas with CBFPS village distributors*			*Control areas*			
	Percentage pregnant Jan 1975*	*Percentage pregnant* Jan 1977*	*Percentage decline*	*Percentage pregnant* Jan 1975*	*Percentage pregnant* Jan 1977*	*Percentage decline*	*Percentage difference CBFPS and control areas*
North	8.4	4.9	42.7	9.1	7.7	15.4	27.3
Central	13.4	7.2	46.3	17.5	14.2	18.9	27.4
North East	15.0	8.3	45.6	17.5	10.9	37.7	7.9
South	17.2	13.0	24.4	11.4	15.0	+31.6	56.0
All regions	13.7	8.2	**40.2**	15.0	11.9	**20.7**	**19.5**

* Married women aged 15–44 years were asked: 'Are you pregnant or do you think you are pregnant?'

Clinically, no major problems were reported by the supervisory doctors and complaints over side-effects have been few. One in 400 felt the programme was 'against religion' or against Thai culture and 1 in 200 said CBFPS was a foreign, imperialist plot.

As a result of decisions taken outside the country, the institutional programme was not as strongly supported as the village programme. Nevertheless, it made a nationwide impact and 320 000 have been instructed in the philosophy of family planning and given the opportunity of receiving contraceptives through reliable, cheap, accessible channels. With the backing of the Teachers' Council a mail order system has been set up supplying approximately 20 000 teachers. In Thailand teachers are often brought to Bangkok, or provincial capitals, during school vacations for refresher courses. At these gatherings, which may involve 1000 teachers, time has been made available for lectures in family planning, followed by the immediate distribution of contraceptives. Valuable data on achieved family size, contraceptive practice and fertility goals has been collected at these meetings and the opportunity given for long term association between teachers and CBFPS, both as distributors and consumers.

In developing countries, school teachers, particularly at the rural level, enjoy higher social status than in the West. Many teachers are married women in the years of maximum fertility and the strategy of meeting their contraceptive needs first has proved sound. Having gained their confidence, they become ideal distributors with links to the rest of the community, usually knowing the parents of their pupils and having a good insight into surrounding social problems.

The private sector programme distributed condoms in urban areas and established family planning depots or 'supermarkets' at major bus terminals in Bangkok. By 1977 the programme distributed twice as many condoms as the Ministry of Public Health and by 1978 was breaking even with the commercial market (Table 3). The private sector programme also plays an important fund-raising role, not only selling contraceptives, but T-shirts, panties, and other products.

Towards self-sufficiency

From the outset the programme was designed to be partially self-sufficient. The largest single group of workers – the village distributors – are remunerated entirely from contraceptive sales. In addition, 80% of the selling price returns directly to the programme and ultimately village districts produce sufficient income to cover running costs and pay back most of the start-up

TABLE 3 Condom distribution by the Ministry of Public Health, the Community-Based Family Planning Service agency (CBFPS) and the commercial companies in Thailand, 1975–77

Year	Condom distribution							
	Ministry of Public Health		*CBFPS*		*Commercial*		*Total*	
	No. (gross)	*% increase*	*No. (gross)*	*% increase*	*No. (gross)*	*% increase*	*No. (gross)*	*% increase*
1975	19 700	—	5080	—	65 000	—	89 780	—
1976	25 433	29%	35 525	70 000	8%	130 958	46%	
1977	36 000	42%	72 273	103%	95 000	36%	203 273	55%

Sources: Family Health Division, Department of Health, Ministry of Public Health 1978
Office of Community-Based Family Planning Services, Bangkok, Thailand, 1978
Marketing survey in Thailand, Durex Company, 1978

costs (Figure 1). Local income now provides more than two thirds of the total budget (Table 4). The private sector programme produces funds from contraceptive sales while fulfilling its prime service and informational role. T-shirts with a variety of designs and slogans have proved popular. It has been cheaper to manufacture these than to have them printed for resale and a small export trade is building up.

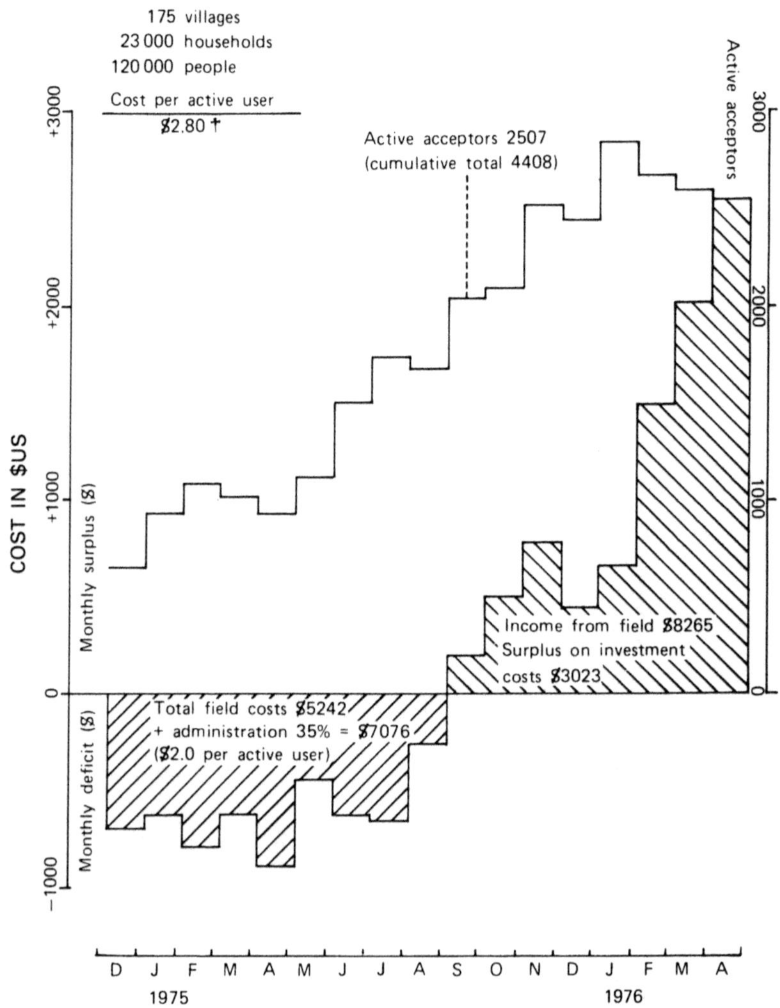

Figure 1 Investment costs, surpluses and number of acceptors for one district
† Seventeen months' programme experience (commodities supplied free of charge)

TABLE 4 Source of funds 1974–77 ($US)

Source	*1974* *Amount*	%	*1975* *Amount*	%	*1976* *Amount*	%	*1977* *Amount*	%	*Grand total 1974–77* *Amount*	%
IPPF grant	235 000	89	275 000	71	260 000	46	174 527	29	944 527	55
Local income	30 500	11	111 769	29	305 769	54	332 309	71	780 402	45
Total	265 500	100	386 769	100	565 769	100	506 836	100	1 724 874	100

In turn these endeavours have created some rather special job opportunities. In their work in the community the CBFPS team inevitably meet cases where unwanted pregnancy has occurred, termination has proved unobtainable and a pregnant (usually unmarried) girl needs support until delivery of the child and its possible adoption. Cases such as these are happily accepted into the CBFPS community and given small jobs from preparing food to printing T-shirts and in some ways the headquarters has become an extended family.

Administration

The span between orchestrating the publicity which is an essential element in successful family planning and organizing the logistics of a service programme covering millions of people who live in the rural sector of a developing country is a large one. The programme is run with an average of 1.2 paid staff per 70 000 population. One of the most important aspects has been the demonstration that it is possible to recruit and train large numbers of distributors and establish a programme that can be replicated rapidly over large areas of a developing country, once the initial structure has been tested. In the first year 24 districts were opened up but three years later 20 new districts were opened in a single month. There seems no reason why similar programmes should not be begun in other countries.

A compact, increasingly cost-effective, central professional staff has been built up. The administrative structure has been analysed and reported by the Asian Institute of Management, the Harvard School of Public Health and has been used as a teaching model in a number of Thai universities and institutions. Staff experience is shared and opinions sought on new ventures. Staff often eat together and morale is high.

PROBLEMS AND OPPORTUNITIES

The IPPF in making available funding and commodities had to act within its own organizational restraints: it receives its budgets on a year by year basis, mainly from donor governments, and similarly the CBFPS programme has had to make its plans on an annual basis. Inevitably, uncertainty about the following year proved a barrier to progress on a number of occasions.

Communications halfway around the world can be difficult. Sometimes money and commodities did not arrive on time and there were embarrassing cash flow problems at the local level, which disturbed a programme where there is considerable pressure on the local team to achieve good results. In addition, the programme was unlucky in that, for entirely coincidental reasons, there were two changes in the senior management of the relevant department of the IPPF in London within a brief interval: it takes time for a new manager of international programmes to learn about a project in a distant land and mistakes and misjudgements are possible during the harassed period of taking up the reins somebody else has dropped.

Sterilization and abortion

As emphasized, the programme has been about family planning as a whole, not individual methods. It has been the external pressure of Thai law and the bureaucratic compartmentalization of international agencies that limited the initial villages' programme to Pills and condoms. The people and those running the programme would have appreciated a wider choice. Abortion has always been practised by traditional midwives, but is limited by statute law to medical indications. The Government Fourth Plan (1977–82) calls for statute changes 'so that abortion can be legally performed for a number of other valid reasons'.

It was not IPPF policy to include injectable contraceptives (Depo-Provera is popular in Thailand) or sterilization in CBFPS, but in 1977 a pilot project in sterilization was financed by the Rockefeller Foundation. The village distributors in an area of Thailand with 680 000 inhabitants were organized as vasectomy referral agents. In a 14 day campaign 717 men were sterilized in a region where in previous years vasectomies had averaged less than one a week. The campaign demonstrated the value of contraceptive distributors in other areas and as 45% of the families had not used *any* method of family planning previously, it underscored the need for a multiplicity of methods; 42% of distributors believed injectable contraceptives would be popular but the addition of this method has not yet proved possible.

Integrated projects

Integration of family planning with other aspects of health care and community development is a popular policy at a governmental level, but often disappointing in the field. It has proved difficult to get agencies and governmental ministries to share in common projects and at worst 'integration' has become an excuse for doing anything but family planning.

In CBFPS integration has been seen not as something to be attempted from the top down, but as a village policy, and the family planning distributor has become the focus for fertility-related community development. The contraceptive distributor's task, once learnt, is straightforward, yet they become potential village leaders by virtue of the service they give to consumers and their continuous contact with the outside world.

The first and most developed CBFPS integrated programmes involved family planning and parasite control. Distributors have organized stool examination, sanitary education and treatment for intestinal parasites as successfully as they have taken part in family planning. In trial projects financed by the Japanese Organisation for International Cooperation in Family Planning, 78% of children were found to have gut parasites, mostly hookworm. (It has been calculated that the protein loss from the intestines of Thailand due to parasites exceeds the export of protein as beef from New Zealand!)

Parasite control has reinforced the role of distributors as family planning agents and in test areas contraceptive use has jumped 12% over control areas without parasite control. The limitation of this type of integrated programme is the high cost of treatment ($1 for an adult treatment and $0.75 for a child) which must be subsidized at a village level. As an alternative, experiments are being conducted with a traditional antiworming herb called *maluka (Diopyros mollis,* Griff.).

Plans are being developed for a range of additional fertility-related development projects: distributors renting buffalos to acceptors; cooperatives for selling village produce organized by the distributor; and rural credit schemes. A beginning has been made in urban areas with Krung Thai Bank which is circulating family planning piggy banks to encourage child saving and remind people about the economic benefits to the family of fertility control.

CONCLUSIONS

Rural, community-based, family planning services can be set up in a developing country using indigenous personnel assisted by a small well-organized full-time staff.

When it began, the CBFPS programme had a number of controversial elements in it. It required a non-physician distribution of the Pill, involved training village distributors and it was a new and autonomous programme that had to work beside the Ministry of Public Health and the pre-existing family planning association. It is fair to say that the initial authorization for the work was not the most solid; risks were taken. However, with the passage of time and the success of the programme, CBFPS filled a pre-existing gap in services and its relationship with sister organizations matured. The programme complements existing services, as the ability to refer couples for the surgical methods of fertility control demonstrates, and it can be the nucleus for other aspects of health and community development, as the addition of parasite control and evolution of credit systems testifies. Given a policy to sell contraceptives at subsidized prices, it is a programme that can be partially self-sufficient even in poor rural areas.

CBFPS would not have succeeded without the correct degree of administrative leadership and autonomy. It was fortunate in being able to relate to the IPPF donor as partner and not a dependent agency. This has enabled it to establish, or begin to establish, relationships with other international agencies such as USAID, the World Bank, the German government and the Rockefeller Foundation. Equally important, a structure was built up which could carry a pilot project in one small area to a programme of national significance in a mere three years. It is a programme that still has a great deal of work in front of it.

Thailand, like many developing countries, is subject to many socio-economic changes. The CBFPS has not changed fertility patterns alone, but it has accelerated an existing trend in a way which, if successfully adopted elsewhere, will go a great deal of the way to solving the Asian or Latin American population problem.

Bibliography

Burnight, R. G. and Boonlert, Leoprapai (1975). *Attitudes of Rural Thai Women towards Induced Abortion.* (Bangkok: Mahidal University)

Community Based Family Planning Services (1976). *First Round of the Household Survey to Evaluate the Effectiveness of CBFPS in Thailand.* (Bangkok: CBFPS)

Rosenfield A. G. and Charoon, Limcharoen (1972). Auxiliary midwife prescription of oral contraceptives. *Am. J. Obstet. Gynecol.,* **114,** 942

Somsak, Varakamin and Debhanom, Muangam (1977). *Seminar on the Progress of Family Planning and the Use of Paramedical Personnel in Family Planning Services.* (Duplicated document)

Warren, W. (1978). Mechai – Thailand's ubiquitous family planner. *Reader's Digest* (Asian edition). **January,** 96

de Yong, J. (1966). *Village Life in Thailand.* (Berkeley: University of California Press)

6

Involving the community – Howrah

Pouru Bhiwandiwala

INTRODUCTION	94
HOWRAH CBD–A BEGINNING	95
Background	95
Delivery system	96
Community involvement	97
Contraceptive method	98
OPERATION OF THE PROJECT	100
Depot holder	101
Follow-up and referral	102
Supervision	103
Depot and supplies	103
REPORTING AND EVALUATION	104
THE ECONOMIC ASPECTS	106
Free versus payment	107
Towards self-sufficiency	108
OVERCOMING BARRIERS AND BOTTLENECKS	109
WHAT LIES AHEAD?	111
Additional options	111
Integration	112
Replicability	113
SHORTCOMINGS AND STRENGTHS	113

INTRODUCTION

In recent years, several innovative programmes have been implemented in a variety of settings with the objective of taking family planning to the world's poor. It is now widely recognized that the physician-oriented or clinic-based system cannot provide this basic need to the hundreds of millions of people who live in rural and relatively isolated regions. The subsequent exploration of various non-clinical delivery systems has clearly demonstrated that the involvement of the community in providing its own services can be most effective. The use of local resources has not only overcome the serious shortage of medical professionals, but has significantly increased the acceptability of family planning. It is often stated that contraceptive use is dependent upon education, employment status, socio-economic level and other factors. However, from a practical point of view, it will be a long time before these conditions are remedied in developing countries, and will continue to contribute to an increase in the number of the world's poor. This vicious cycle must be broken, and there is sufficient international evidence to indicate that the system of community-based distribution of contraceptives can overcome these factors.

India is facing a population explosion of crisis dimensions which has largely diluted the fruits of the economic progress that has been made over the last two decades. The population now stands at 620 million, and if the current growth rate continues the country will reach the 1 billion mark by the end of the century. There are approximately 21 million births and 8 million deaths annually, thereby adding 13 to 14 million to the existing population every year. With only 2.4% of the world's land area and 2% of the total world income, India supports 15% of the world's population. The rapid decline in the death rate without a concomitant decline in the birth rate has produced a rapidly growing population in an already highly populated country.

The unprecedented growth has staggered the imagination of policy planners attempting to provide food, shelter, clothing, education, jobs, health care and cremation facilities. In order to provide for the annual population increase of 13 million, India has to find every year an additional 12 545 300 quintals of food; 188 774 000 metres of cloth; 126 500 additional schools; 372 500 additional teachers; 2 509 000 houses and 4 000 000 new jobs – a prospect which would daunt even the most affluent country.

Recognizing the high fertility rate and rapid population growth as major obstacles to the country's socio-economic progress, in 1952 the government of India adopted a comprehensive family planning policy as an integral part of its national development plans. Unfortunately, the facilities were mainly located in urban areas and larger towns, which were inaccessible to those who most needed the services. About 81.9% of India's population lives in 557 989 villages scattered all over the country. Major transportation and communication difficulties exist in reaching many of these villages. By 1964, when the situation had become a matter of national survival, the government decided to extend the family planning programme to the rural areas, by integrating it with the existing health services.

A network of Primary Health Centres (PHCs) supported by the government is supposed to provide basic preventive and curative health care to the rural population. Each PHC caters to 100 000 people, but in practice it is not accessible to all the villagers due to lack of transport. The supply of contraceptives, when available, is often intermittent and erratic, depending upon the resources, weather and availability of personnel. By adding family planning to an already inadequate infrastructure, the demand for family planning services in the rural areas remains largely unmet.

HOWRAH CBD – A BEGINNING

Background

Howrah is an extremely poor district in the state of West Bengal, with a population of 2.6 million. It consists essentially of rural areas but includes what may well be the world's poorest slum on the outskirts of Calcutta. The living conditions and transportation system leave much to be desired; the housing ranges from poorly constructed brick structures to shanty huts put together with makeshift materials. Sanitation is almost non-existent, and the water supply is generally obtained from a local well. During the monsoon season, it is frequently necessary for people to wade kneedeep through water to enter their homes. Overcrowding is usual, and it is not uncommon to find animals too sharing the same dwelling.

Roads and public transport do not exist in many areas of Howrah. In fact, the only access to some of the remote regions in this district is by boat. Bullock-carts, bicycles, cycle rickshaws and palanquins (a covered seat carried on poles on the shoulders of two or four men) are commonly used modes of transport. But by and large the villagers depend on their own two feet.

It is estimated that of the 2.6 million people living in Howrah, about 390 000 couples are in the fertile age group. Survey data on these eligible couples are currently being analysed, and were not available at the time of writing. However, it is apparent that the typical characteristics of the rural population in India are equally true for Howrah – low literacy and socioeconomic levels, early marriages, large family-size norms and high infant mortality. Yet for most of these people, according to Potts, 'access to modern contraceptives is as remote as the possibility of going to university; and the option of the surgical means of fertility control as unlikely as owning a car'.

Under these adverse and difficult conditions, a community-based project was launched in Howrah to distribute oral contraceptives as widely as possible among the eligible couples in this district. In addition to the service component of this programme, there is a built-in evaluation system to determine its safety, cost-effectiveness and capability of producing a demographic impact. This project was initiated by the International Fertility Research Program) (IFRP), Research Triangle Park, North Carolina, using funds made available by the Population Crisis Committee, Washington, DC. It is currently being monitored and evaluated by the India Fertility Research Programme with technical support from the IFRP.

Delivery system

The Howrah CBD Project materialized on the assumption that non-availability rather than lack of motivation was the major barrier to contraceptive acceptance. Although the villagers are illiterate, they are at the same time fairly intelligent. There was every reason to believe that if the means of regulating their fertility was made available to them they would certainly use it. On questioning the people, it was evident that community participation and involvement in providing their own services would be forthcoming.

The Howrah district consists of 26 Community Development Blocks (administrative units in rural areas), with an approximate population of 100 000 in each block. In order to facilitate the implementation of this village-based project, each of these blocks is further divided into ten Depot Distribution Units (10 000 population), with a Contraceptive Supply Depot in each unit. A total of 260 such depots is expected to cover the entire population of Howrah.

The Contraceptive Supply Depot is staffed by a depot holder (preferably a female) who is selected from the local community, and given the necessary training. She visits, motivates and registers all the eligible couples in her geographical area of responsibility, and this process is considerably simplified as she already knows most of the people. The depot is kept open for a fixed period of time every day (generally 2 to 3 hours), 6 days a week; the women are requested to come at this time for their supply of Pills. The depot holder maintains a simple record on each woman, and obtains a medical history at the time of the first visit. If there are no contraindications (which are specified on a checklist), the depot holder will dispense the oral contraceptives and provide the necessary advice and instructions. In the event of a doubtful or evident contraindication, the woman is referred to the Primary Health Centre or a local doctor if available. In order to ensure adequate follow-up and effectively deal with any side-effects, only one cycle of Pills is supplied at each visit. A simple and practical tickler system is maintained by the depot holder in order to follow up the acceptors. If a woman fails to come to the depot for 3 days after the scheduled visit for resupply, the depot holder visits her and investigates the cause for the delay.

For every ten depots, one supervisor is appointed to assist the depot holders in all aspects of their work, ensure that they are performing their duties satisfactorily, and provide onsite training as necessary. The supervisors report to the Project Director at the Headquarters Office. This office is responsible for the management of the programme and a major administrative function is to ensure that all depots are adequately stocked with contraceptives.

Community involvement

Although the Howrah CBD Project began from a different starting point than the one in Thailand (described in Chapter 5), a key element of both programmes is that they build on the social structure of the communities they serve. The political and social acceptability of the programme is enhanced by using local resources, and making the community members a part of the delivery system. The Howrah Project takes maximum advantage of the commonsense, goodwill and existing skills of the villagers; and the response has been most rewarding. Before initiating any activities in a village, the Project Director and his staff first explain the programme to the local community leaders and enlist their support. A Community Advisory Committee is formed and the membership consists of the village and religious leaders, traditional practitioners, holy men and representatives from local social organizations (particularly women's groups and youth associations). The main function of this committee is to actually implement the CBD system in their village (or group of villages), with the assistance of the regional supervisor and Headquarters Office Staff. The committee members tend to take this responsibility seriously, as there is a certain degree of competition between villages, and each committee tries to outdo the other.

One of the earlier tasks performed by the committee is the selection of the depot holder from the local community. The Project Director and supervisor provide the members with guidelines and selection criteria, but the ultimate choice is entirely up to the committee. This has invariably resulted in the selection of a person who is accepted by the entire community. The next step is to provide a centrally located depot for the storage and distribution of the Pills. As the budget for this programme does not allow any rental or maintenance for depots (and this is deliberate), it necessarily involves the use of local village resources. Although the Community Advisory Committee serves many important functions, its most significant role is that it lends respectability to the programme and dramatically increases its acceptability. The villagers will wholeheartedly accept an idea which has been blessed, endorsed and implemented by their own leaders. In every sense, the Community Advisory Committee is vital for the success of the programme, as the members understand the local customs and attitudes, and their recommendations are of much greater value than those of the experts or consultants.

The inauguration of a depot is a community event, and it is usually marked by a grand and colourful opening ceremony. The villagers turn up in all their finery; the leaders deliver speeches emphasizing their support to the Project; and the first few women enrolled in the Project have the privilege of publicly receiving their initial supply of Pills from the Chief Guest – a process which is accompanied by considerable applause from the audience. Refreshments are served and some enterprising groups may even provide entertainment. Everybody is very happy, and the CBD Project is off to a good start.

As the Howrah Project basically relies on local community resources (other than the supply of pills), this minimizes the chances of disruption of services due to external factors. The depot holder's task of motivating the couples is considerably simplified, as the awareness among the community has already been created. Since the whole village has accepted the idea, the use of contraception can be discussed openly and freely. There is no need for secrecy, as the fear of negative reactions from relatives and friends has been eliminated. Satisfied users readily pass the word around, and this serves as the most effective motivating force. The depot holder is able to approach the family as a unit, and avoid the disparity between husband and wife regarding family-size norms.

Contraceptive method

Any programme has to be based on a contraceptive method and a distribution system. Even though the so-called 'cafeteria' approach is considered to be the ideal situation, it is not always possible to implement. Additional options would be highly desirable, but out of necessity the Howrah Project has currently been restricted to a single contraceptive method. Although the Indian government does not promote the use of oral contraceptives in the National Family Planning Programme, consideration of several factors led to the decision of using Pills as the method of choice. Oral contraceptives have been thoroughly evaluated and proven effective, safe and appropriate for use by poor and illiterate women. Also, the experience of using paramedical workers to distribute Pills and provide follow-up for acceptors has been most satisfactory. This method also eliminates the need for clinical services (except as a back-up), and the costs are acceptable.

Oral contraceptives have a much worse public image than they deserve, as it has been conclusively shown that they represent an acceptable risk level when compared to the alternative of unwanted pregnancy, particularly in developing countries. Although it is not possible to guarantee the safety of administering Pills in a non-clinical setting, the Howrah Project has taken every possible precaution (within its limitations) to maximize the safety and effectiveness. During the training of the depot holder, considerable emphasis is placed on the proper selection of Pill users. The depot holder is required to obtain a detailed medical history for every woman who is registered in the programme. In order to simplify this process, a special checklist of contra-indications is printed on the *couple registration form* (Table 1) which is completed by the depot holder before dispensing pills to any woman.

TABLE 1 Couple registration form

MEDICAL HISTORY

Check (√) appropriate answer

Does the woman currently have:

	No	Yes
1. Yellow skin or eyes		
2. Breast mass(es)		
3. Watery or bloody discharge from the breast (nipple)		
4. Abnormal menstrual periods or frequent vaginal bleeding		
5. Vaginal bleeding after intercourse		
6. Swollen and/or painful legs		
7. Severe chest pain		
8. Weakness or shortness of breath after exertion		
9. Frequent, severe headaches		
10. Varicose veins		
11. An infant three months old or less whom she is breastfeeding		
12. Is the woman over 35 years old and does she smoke cigarettes		

If a positive response is obtained for any of these conditions, the woman is referred to the nearest Primary Health Centre or physician.

Several serious side-effects are known to occur with the use of oral contraceptives, but it must be emphasized that the risk/benefit ratio varies considerably by country and age-group. The rural women in developing countries are less prone to various medical disabilities which contraindicate Pills (such as thromboembolic disorders and hypertension), and the alarm over side-effects with the use of Pills has been grossly exaggerated. The health hazards associated with pregnancy and labour in this population of women far outweigh the potential risks of morbidity and mortality in Pill-users. The complaints of minor side-effects is extremely low amongst these women, essentially because of their high tolerance developed by living in such a difficult environment. It is the author's experience that even on making positive suggestions, the women did not appear to be bothered by the minor symptoms, and considered these, if any, to have a relatively negligible nuisance value as compared to the burden of annual childbearing.

By assessing the relevant benefits and risks of Pills, and by taking into account the underlying characteristics of the Howrah population, the demographic factors, social customs and nature of the health delivery system, there was enough evidence to indicate that the Pill would be a suitable contraceptive method.

OPERATION OF THE PROJECT

The Howrah CBD Project is the first of its kind in India, and therefore in addition to the service component, it has a built-in ongoing evaluation system. It is hoped that the data will prove useful not only in measuring the effectiveness of the programme, but will also serve to identify areas requiring improvement, and determine the replicability of the project in other regions of India. Accordingly, the objectives of this programme are:

* To distribute oral contraceptives at a reasonable cost as widely as possible among the eligible couples in Howrah district. (Total number of eligible couples: 390 000; target number of couples: 150 000.)
* To evaluate the delivery system in order to maximize the cost-effectiveness and efficiency without sacrificing the quality of the services.
* To analyse programme impact through an assessment of:
  (a) the prevalence of contraceptive practice attributable to the programme;
  (b) the number of couple-years of protection provided by the programme;
  (c) any fertility change that takes place in the district, and the effect that the Community-Based Distribution Programme may have had on that change.
* To determine the replicability of the Project in other regions of India.

Depot holder

The entire CBD Project evolves around the depot holders, and it is the collective performance of these individuals that will ultimately determine the outcome of the programme. It is therefore understandable why such considerable importance is placed on the selection and training of the volunteers, who will serve their respective communities as depot holders. The guidelines for identifying such a person are quite flexible, and the choice is left entirely to the discretion of the local Community Advisory Committee. The depot holder is preferably a woman with a high-school education which would enable her to maintain simple records and service statistics. Some experience in social work is desirable but not necessary. The profession of the volunteer is not a major consideration in the selection process, and experience has shown that housewives have the maturity, motivation and family life to do an excellent job. However, the essential criteria for qualifying as a depot holder are that the person must be from the local village or group of villages, and should have sufficient standing and respect in the community.

There is considerable variation in the literature regarding the duration and magnitude of training that needs to be provided to distributors of contraceptives. It ranges from the sublimely simple (even monkeys can be trained to distribute pills!) to intensive training in several aspects of family planning. The Howrah Project skirts around this problem by dividing the training into three phases: initial instruction at the Head Office, supplemented by field training on home grounds provided by the supervisor, and finally a refresher or retraining course about 3 to 6 months later. The depot holder gains an understanding about the working of the distribution system, family planning education and motivation, the use of oral contraceptives (including contraindications and side-effects), interviewing techniques, depot management, record keeping, and client referral procedures. Some volunteers initially work as an assistant to a depot holder in an adjoining group of villages, till they have acquired sufficient experience to establish a depot in their own community.

The depot holder performs two major functions – education, motivation and follow-up of eligible couples; and maintenance of a depot for Pill supplies and distribution. She systematically visits the eligible couples, and it generally takes several months to cover the entire geographical area of her responsibility. She registers each of these couples, questions them about their desire for additional children and motivates them to accept family planning. In addition to visiting each household, the depot holder also meets and talks to groups of men at work. A good place to get a captive audience of women is at the local village well which is the only source of water supply, and is visited daily by most women. This provides a venue for discussion and sharing of experiences amongst the women, and reassurance from satisfied Pill users appears to be the most effective mechanism for increasing the number of acceptors. The depot holder also meets groups of women working in the fields, at the local weaving and spinning centre, and other sites where women are employed in cottage industries. This dual approach enables the couples to get the individual attention of the depot holder when she visits them at home, and they also have the opportunity of discussing this matter with other members of their own sex when the depot holder approaches them in groups.

Although motivation forms an important aspect of the depot holder's duties, the voluntary nature of this programme is strongly and constantly emphasized. The depot holder is strictly forbidden to use pressure tactics to influence the decision of any couple. If the woman is willing to accept contraception, she is requested to come to the depot for her supply of Pills. If she is uncertain, the depot holder will visit her again after some time.

Follow-up and referral

The depot holder is instructed to maintain a balance between her efforts to enrol new clients and maintain a good follow-up of the acceptors. This is partly accomplished by the fact that only one cycle of Pills is provided to the women, and so they have to visit the depot monthly for supplies. The side-effects are promptly treated, and anxiety, if any, is allayed. These frequent visits also ensure continuous interaction, motivation and encouragement, all of which contribute significantly to an increased contraceptive continuation rate. The depot holder is required to call on every client who misses her scheduled visit to the depot by three days, in order to investigate the cause of the delay. If the missed appointment is due to negligence, the depot holder invariably expresses her resentment and strongly discourages a repetition.

Prior to the Pill distribution in any community, arrangements are always made for a reliable back-up source. Wherever available, the local doctor generally agrees to assume this responsibility, and in other communities the depot holder may have to rely on the Primary Health Centre in spite of the distance. However, the bulk of the referrals are made to three clinics in Howrah which provide family planning services, such as IUD insertions, menstrual regulation procedures and management of side-effects associated with the Pill. Each of these clinics is a simple one-room facility which operates for 2 days a week, and is managed by a visiting doctor from Calcutta and an assistant. For women requesting sterilization, the nearest services available are in the neighbouring city of Calcutta. Although every effort is made to provide a reasonable back-up, it must be admitted that there are several remote communities where the women would have to travel an extensive distance in order to avail themselves of these services.

Supervision

The extent of supervision currently varies among different communities, but the Project aims to provide one supervisor for every ten depots. The supervisors are generally recruited from two categories of personnel – a depot holder who has demonstrated outstanding merit, or a previous government-employed community health worker. Unlike the new depot holders, these individuals have extensive practical experience in community work. This is further supplemented by training at the Head Office prior to assuming their duties.

The supervisor reports to the Project Director and maintains a liaison between the field and the Head Office. His primary function is to supervise the depot holders, and provide guidance and advice. He is also responsible for setting up a depot and conducting onsite training for the new depot holder. He routinely inspects the records maintained by the depot holders, and periodically prepares status reports which summarize this information. The supervisor frequently checks the inventory maintained by the depot holder to ensure that an adequate reserve of contraceptive supplies is always available.

In order to assess the quality of the services provided to the community, the supervisor visits acceptors at random and interviews them. Any irregularities or problems are thereby brought to his attention, and this enables him to take the necessary action to upgrade the services. A new depot holder is very carefully and closely monitored, but after the programme is well-established in the community, the supervisor plays more of an advisory role and it is the depot holder who actually runs the show.

Depot and supplies

Setting up a depot is entirely a community effort, and the ingenuity of the villagers in providing a suitable place is absolutely fascinating. As mentioned earlier in the chapter, not a single cent is budgeted for the rental, maintenance or repair of the depot, and this responsibility rests solely with the community. The size, condition and appearance of the depot is irrelevant, but the two important requirements are that it must be located within walking distance of the majority of the village population, and it should be available for the specified period of time every day. So far, this has not posed a problem in any of the villages where the programme is ongoing. A variety of sites have been used to set up depots, and these include the village meeting-place, classroom, library, shed, unoccupied house, storage room, etc. In a Muslim community, the village leaders have donated the use of a room which is an extension of the mosque.

These depots are basically simple shelters with no additional facilities, and the depot holder is perfectly content if she has a table and chair. The grounds outside serve as a waiting-room, and very often the depot holder also prefers to work in the open air. No matter how simple and meagre the facilities, the large prominent signboard outside each depot immediately lends it respectability.

At the conclusion of her training at the Head Office, the depot holder returns to her village with all the essential supplies. These include a strong metal trunk to store the contraceptives, a signboard for the depot, pamphlets to be used for information and motivation, forms and registers for record-keeping, and of course, a generous supply of oral contraceptives. Plastic ziplock bags are also supplied for dispensing the Pill packets to provide protection against moisture and heat. These bags have proved to be extremely popular among the local population, and it is amazing to note the number of ways in which they are subsequently used. Each depot holder is presented with an impressive shoulderbag, on which the family planning symbol and name of the Project is imprinted. She uses it to store her materials during home visits, and it also serves to draw attention to her message. In addition to being a practical item, the depot holder is proud to carry it around as a status-symbol.

REPORTING AND EVALUATION

The record-keeping system for this Project is somewhat elaborate and time-consuming, but it must be recognized that the CBD programme is the very first of its kind in India, and needs to be thoroughly evaluated in order to determine its effectiveness. In the present system, the major responsibility for maintaining records is placed on the depot holder. She is required to complete a *couple registration record* for each eligible couple whom she has interviewed in her area. This includes identification of the couple and depot holder, and information on couple characteristics such as age, parity, the wife's pregnancy status, and any contraceptive method the couple may have used in the last three months before contact. The next section deals with programme participation and calls for information on the contraceptive supplied to the couple and reason for referral if any. The medical history consists of a checklist of contraindications (relative and absolute) to oral contraceptives. This couple registration record serves as a permanent record, and all of the follow-up data on complaints, referrals, number of Pill cycles supplied and reasons for discontinuation are recorded on the back of this form.

When a woman receives her first cycle of Pills, she is also given an identification card. Instructions for the use of oral contraceptives are printed on the back of this card in the local language. The depot holder records each supply visit on this card, and notes the date for the client's next visit. As a tickler system for follow-up, the depot holder uses a regular desk diary. She enters the name and couple registration number of the woman on the date on which her next visit has been scheduled. Every day the depot holder checks off the names of the women who have reported to the depot for supplies. If a woman fails to arrive, she is given 3 days' grace, after which the depot holder will visit her at home and investigate the cause for the delay.

The depot holder also maintains a daily register in which she enters the client's name, couple registration number, date of visit, Pill cycles supplied, the client's programme status and any referral made. The client is requested to sign the register or affix her thumbprint to acknowledge receiving the Pills. At the end of each month, the depot holder prepares a summary card which indicates the number of couples interviewed, new acceptors, Pill cycles distributed and the stock position. This is sent to the Head Office, and the information is used to monitor the depot holder's activities, as well as ensure that there is no breakdown in contraceptive supplies. In addition, the supervisor (with the assistance of the depot holder) prepares a status report every 6 months for the respective time-period. This is based on information from the couple registration records (including the follow-up section), for either all or a sample of the programme participants comprising of previous, new and reactivated acceptors.

The strength of this record-keeping system lies in its ability to provide a feedback on several aspects of programme performance and management. The service statistics can be obtained by a combination of manual and computer tabulations. A certain degree of flexibility does exist, and the system can be adapted to meet special needs in a variety of settings. It can be supplemented with contraceptive prevalence surveys to obtain information on eligible couples who do not participate in the programme; to determine the traditional methods of fertility control being used by the community; to pinpoint problems in areas of poor performance; and finally to assess the impact of the programme on contraceptive use and ultimately on fertility rates.

An analysis of the couple registration records will provide a 'survey of eligible couples' for the geographical area of each depot, and this data can be pooled to provide statistics for the entire Howrah district. The information thus generated will include the socio-demographic characteristics of eligible couples, their family patterns, desire for additional children, and history of contraceptive use. It will also be possible to compare the characteristics of couples who accept oral contraceptives with those who do not, in order to identify 'high risk couples', and assess the impact of the Project. Analysis of the data on the Status Reports will yield important indices related to programme performance such as participation status, continuation rates, reasons for discontinuation, patterns of contraceptive use, couple-years of protection, failure rates, and the number of Pill cycles distributed. Maximum emphasis will be placed on the continuation rates, as an indicator to assess the Project's effectiveness.

After the programme has been adequately evaluated and redirected wherever necessary, the record-keeping will be considerably simplified. (It is an accepted fact that 10%, or even less, of the records kept world-wide are ever used.) Limited information will be collected to serve two essential purposes. First, the depot holders will require a system to define the local targets and ensure systematic coverage of their areas; second, the progress of the Project will be monitored essentially based on numerical achievements. This could be accomplished either by a sample survey or computerization of a simple record system. It is yet to be conclusively established as to which of these methods would be cheaper and easier to implement.

THE ECONOMIC ASPECTS

Since family planning must reach hundreds of millions of people, the economic considerations are of paramount importance. Most programme managers are critically assessing the cost-effectiveness, and exploring means to achieve at least partial self-sufficiency. Although it is acknowledged that innovative pilot projects are likely to be more expensive than large well-established traditional programmes, it has been demonstrated that most community-based projects have proved to be significantly cheaper and more effective in the long term. There is a definite trend towards using a plurality of monetary systems, whereby the programme participants are required to make a partial contribution towards the cost of the contraceptive, but at the same time the totally indigent receive the services entirely free. Likewise the distributors range from volunteers who do not get any financial remuneration, to those who are paid salaries or receive a commission based on the sales and/or distribution.

The Howrah Project operates on an annual budget of $50 000, but this does *not* include the cost of the oral contraceptives which have been donated by an international agency. It must be pointed out that all the depots (total, 260) are provided and maintained by the local communities. Not a single cent is spent on construction or heavy capital investments. The depot holder does not receive a salary, but in addition to the non-monetary incentives of prestige and recognition, she obtains a decent income from two sources. The acceptors are charged Rs. 0.25 (approximately 3 US cents) for each cycle of pills, and the depot holder is allowed to retain this payment. It is estimated that a fully operational depot should have an average of 500 acceptors, which amounts to a fairly significant monthly income for the depot holder. In addition, she is paid Rs. 0.75 (approximately 9 US cents) for every couple registration record, which she completes at the time of interviewing the couple and periodically submits to the Head Office. There is a tendency among some depot holders to concentrate more on filling in this record rather than following up users, as it is financially more rewarding. This has been counteracted to some extent by placing a limit of 125 couple registration records which may be completed each month. It is interesting to note that some enthusiastic and aggressive depot holders have employed an assistant, who is paid from their own personal income, to help with the increasing workload.

The current cost per acceptor per annum is approximately $2.00 excluding the cost of the Pills, but this is expected to decrease to about US $0.50 to $0.75 per acceptor per annum towards the end of the 2 year period, when the target number of 150 000 acceptors has been achieved. This compares quite favourably with other ongoing community programmes.

Enlightened donors can contribute significantly to the success of a project. It must be stated to the eternal credit of the Population Crisis Committee in Washington, DC, that senior members of the agency had the courage and foresight to invest their funds in a risky, innovative project. Furthermore, they did not impose any regulations, beyond the simple requirement of periodic financial and progress reports. The encouragement and interest of the donors, combined with their tolerance and flexibility have served to convert a concept into a reality.

Free versus payment

There is a considerable difference of opinion regarding payment for contraceptives, and the options include free, subsidized and at-cost distribution, and finally commercial marketing for profit. It is generally accepted that a nominal amount should be charged, so that the user credits the contraceptive with more value and effectiveness, and the probability of use is higher. This also serves to reduce the financial demand on the programme and assures ultimate self-sufficiency. Another merit of charging for services is that it is an excellent means of rewarding the field staff in a way that is difficult to corrupt. For instance, in the Howrah Project the depot holder keeps the payment for the contraceptives, and this acts as a most effective incentive since her income is directly proportional to her efforts. Furthermore, the depot holder has nothing to gain by falsifying the records or number of acceptors, as her earnings depend entirely on the payment she receives from the contraceptive users. Another welcome side-effect is that the depot holder will go to great lengths to ensure that she has an adequate stock of contraceptives, and a breakdown in the supply pipeline is less likely.

Although most programme managers acknowledge the advantages of charging for services, they unanimously and strongly feel that contraceptives must be distributed entirely free of cash payment, to the totally indigent who want to use them. A major drawback of the Howrah Project is that it lacks such a provision. It is true that the amount charged for the Pills is nominal, and does not pose a financial strain on most of the couples. But in any population, there are always some families who have to choose between food and a cycle of Pills, and no programme can be considered to be totally successful unless it caters to the needs of the poorest.

Towards self-sufficiency

Most family planning programmes have to depend on a substantial input of funds from external sources, particularly during the initial phase. However, it is unrealistic to rely solely on outside support, as the currently available resources for family planning (see Chapters 15 and 16), are totally inadequate to meet the demands. Nor is it likely that the major international donors will significantly increase their contributions in the near future. Limited resources coupled with the problem of galloping inflation, make it mandatory for every programme to seek some level of local funding. The need to focus on the issue of self-sufficiency as an essential long-range programme requirement cannot be overstated. While it may not be possible for every programme to rapidly achieve a status of financial independence, the process can certainly be accelerated by further developing commercial marketing of contraceptives; involving the private sector; promoting the indigenous manufacture of contraceptive commodities; increasing availability of sterilization (which is a most cost-effective method); and finally, developing local technical expertise supplemented by consultant services when required.

In designing the Howrah Project, considerable thought has been given to this aspect of the planning. It is estimated that in three years, the project will yield a reasonable income thus reducing the extent of outside support, and at the end of the 5-year period it should be totally self-sufficient (including the cost of the contraceptives). As mentioned earlier, the contraceptive users are currently paying Rs. 0.25 (3 US cents) for a cycle of Pills; after the depot is well-established, the price will be increased to Rs. 0.50 (6 US cents). The depot holder continues to keep Rs. 0.25 as compensation for her services, and she turns over the remaining amount to the Head Office. This increment has already been implemented in a few depots. There was some initial resistance by the depot holders who even threatened to go on strike, but there was no disruption of services. By and large, the villagers accepted this very philosophically, and the continuation rates as well as recruitment of new acceptors were not affected.

The Project Director is currently exploring the feasibility of tableting and packaging the oral contraceptives locally, and maintaining a good quality control. It is estimated that the actual cost of each Pill cycle could be reduced to about 4 US cents. This is definitely an important step towards ultimate self-sufficiency. Plans are underway for making voluntary sterilization services periodically available, probably with the help of a visiting team. Another significant step is that the responsibility for management and evaluation has been transferred to the local staff, and now IFRP essentially functions in an advisory and consultant capacity. In order for the programme to achieve total self-sufficiency, the cost of the Pills will be gradually increased in stages, till it reaches the amount of Rs. 1 (12 US cents) per cycle. The depot holder will retain her share of Rs. 0.25, and the remainder will cover the actual cost of the Pills and overhead expenses.

OVERCOMING BARRIERS AND BOTTLENECKS

It is commonly presumed that the major barrier in taking family planning to the world's poor lies in their lack of motivation and response. Illiteracy, religion, culture and the poor mother-in-law have all shared the blame for the so-called *resistance* to fertility control. It is acknowledged that these factors along with traditional social norms (need for sons, children to provide social security, etc.) are partly responsible for creating a bottleneck, but they are not unsurmountable. According to Dr Ravenholt, 'contraceptive availability at the household or village level has been demonstrated to override educational, occupational, economic and religious barriers to contraceptive use'. The Howrah CBD Project is essentially based on this conviction, and the receptivity of the villagers has clearly shown that all cultural and religious barriers disappear as the mist before the sun.

Political opposition or indifference poses a serious restraint both on provision of family planning services and acceptance by the potential consumer. Some aspects of family planning remain controversial in several countries. For instance, India has had a National Family Planning Programme since 1952, but even after 26 years of existence, oral contraceptives are still not included. It is believed that the average rural woman is too ignorant to be able to take the Pills correctly, and that it is dangerous to dispense them without medical supervision. It is sincerely hoped that the Howrah Project will successfully explode several myths in this area.

Many a programme has been known to fail because the contraceptives and method of delivery have not been acceptable to the community. It is essential to determine what the people want, and not impose what is supposedly good for them. By involving the community right from the start, the Howrah Project has counteracted any possible resistance from the local practitioners, religious and village leaders. The extent of leadership participation is amply demonstrated by the fact that one of the depots is actually located in the extension of a mosque. The use of a local person to serve as depot holder considerably softens the resistance offered by some traditional communities. In an urban situation, a general and pelvic examination and laboratory investigations are routinely performed prior to dispensing Pills, but this would be totally unacceptable by a rural community. These requirements have therefore been eliminated, and emphasis is placed on a detailed medical history to ensure proper selection of oral contraceptive users. Secretary Gatmaitan (Ministry of Health, the Philippines) has eloquently stated that an acceptable programme is one which 'considers people not merely as targets or numbers to be accounted for, but people who have feelings and emotions that can be hurt, and who have reasons for doing almost anything they do'.

Availability is an important factor which will ultimately determine the effectiveness of the family planning programme. The initial number of new acceptors depends on the motivation, publicity, encouragement from local leadership and widespread distribution of the commodities. However, the continued use of the contraceptives will essentially be determined by knowledge of proper use and constant availability. In Howrah, the major problem of geographic availability has been overcome by setting up depots in each village or group of villages, within walking distance of the local population. This is not only desirable but essential due to the lack of adequate transport, and frequent flooding of the roads. Apart from benefiting the consumers, it also enables the depot holder to visit easily the households in her area of responsibility, to maintain contact with her clients and enrol new acceptors.

The necessity for maintaining an abundant stock of contraceptives both at the depots as well as at the central supply office cannot be overemphasized. The depot holder will not seek new acceptors aggressively, unless she has a substantial supply of commodities to back-up her efforts. Disruption in supply weakens the motivation for continued use as well as discouraging potential clients. The major barrier that the Howrah CBD Project faced a few months ago was a shortage of Pills and subsequent breakdown in the distribution system. Due to various bureaucratic procedures, a large shipment of Pills was unduly delayed, and this proved to be a most serious and costly setback. The opening of several new depots had to be postponed, even though the community was all geared to start. The depot holders were reluctant to recruit new acceptors due to the uncertainty of supplies. The entire momentum was halted, and even though the Pills were available shortly afterwards, it took some time to resume the original pace. However the lesson has been well-learned, and every possible precaution has now been taken to avoid a recurrence. It can be safely stated that, in order to be successful, a programme must be able to assure a supply as well as reliable resupply to the remotest area.

WHAT LIES AHEAD?

Additional options

A drawback of the Howrah Project is that it is based on a single method of contraception. It is obvious that what is acceptable to one couple may be totally unsuitable for another, and this is why the so-called 'cafeteria' approach has emerged. The effectiveness of any family planning programme can be enhanced by making additional options available. Experience has shown that whenever a new method is added, more acceptors are invariably recruited, and the existing methods are not necessarily displaced. Even those who wish to continue with the same method have the satisfaction of making the choice. The necessity for a variety of methods can be compared to means of transportation – in the present jet age, there is a need for the car, bicycle and even an animal-drawn cart.

The Howrah Project has been limited to one method due to necessity rather than preference, and at this stage it would certainly be advantageous to increase the range of options. The methods which would be feasible to introduce at this time are condoms, female barrier methods and Depo-Provera (injectable contraceptive). Due to financial and logistic restraints, these additional methods will only be made available in a few depots, after training the respective depot holders in the use and management of these methods. If the outcome is successful, they will be gradually phased in till all the depots are covered. However, the use of the injectable contraceptive will be restricted to those areas which are adjacent to the Primary Health Centre and the three Howrah clinics.

Integration

There is considerable controversy concerning the value of integrating family planning with health services. This issue will always be difficult to resolve, as both the proponents and opponents extend strong arguments with equal sentiment and passion. It is claimed that family planning would be more acceptable as families prefer a single source of care, and that the programme would substantially benefit from the experience of health personnel and existing facilities. On the other hand, opponents of this theory feel that integration would divert attention from the task of distributing contraceptives and is 'as relevant as attempting to assemble motor cars on a railway station, just because both happen to be means of transport'.

It is obvious that there is no perfect solution, and integration can either enhance or hinder the family planning programme, depending upon the local situation. In order to test the validity of the hypothesis, primary health care services will be introduced in ten depots. An additional ten depots with similar programme duration, contraceptive prevalence and continuation rates will be selected to act as controls. A community survey will be conducted in the experimental area before and some time after introduction of the health care services, in order to evaluate the change, if any, in contraceptive prevalence and continuation rates. A Community Health Volunteer (CHV) will be selected from the villages in each experimental depot area, and will receive special training in the treatment of about ten commonly occurring symptoms (fever, diarrhoea, vomiting, abdominal pain, etc.). No diagnostic skills are involved. The CHV will be provided with a medicine kit, and will administer a drug to treat a specific symptom. If the patient does not respond, or manifests a symptom which is not included in the training of the CHV, he or she is referred to the nearest Primary Health Centre. The CHV will charge about 3 to 6 US cents per treatment.

If the provision of primary health care causes a significant increase in contraceptive acceptance then these services will be gradually extended to other depots. Subsequent introduction of a parasite control programme and immunization are being considered. The results are rapid, visible and beneficial, and if they serve to increase the contraceptive prevalence, it would be a welcome bonus.

Replicability

The Howrah Project has clearly demonstrated that the community-based non-clinical approach has been successful in meeting the family planning needs of a population of 2.6 million in one district of West Bengal. However, there are over 620 million people in India, most of whom live in the rural areas and have limited access to means for controlling their fertility. No doubt there are marked differences in the Indian people, and what holds good in one part of the country may be totally unsuitable elsewhere. But two facts stand out very clearly – the majority of the people in spite of their poverty, illiteracy and social norms *do* want to voluntarily plan their families; and the community-based approach is feasible and practical, and is probably the only way to reach the millions.

It can be stated with reasonable confidence that if a project could be successfully implemented in Howrah with its prevailing difficult conditions, no area in India should be ruled out. Many social, cultural and geographical differences will prevail, but these can be accommodated by suitable variations in the approach. A proposal is currently being considered by the government of India to replicate this project in several states across the country.

SHORTCOMINGS AND STRENGTHS

No project can be absolutely perfect, but the important thing is to recognize and acknowledge the shortcomings, and strive to correct them to the extent possible. Some factors can be remedied and others can only be modified, but considering the overall benefits of a programme, a few deficiencies have to be accommodated. The main drawbacks of the Howrah Project (which have been discussed in various sections of this chapter) are outlined below:

* The entire programme is built on a single contraceptive method, and the consumers have no choice.
* There is no provision for supplying free contraceptives to the totally indigent.
* The record-keeping system is rather elaborate and time-consuming, and detracts from the care provided to contraceptive users.
* Collecting information on eligible couples in the area is financially more rewarding for the depot holder, than following up contraceptive acceptors.
* The referral system is far from adequate. Too much reliance is placed on the already overburdened Primary Health Centre which caters to a population of 100 000 and is staffed by only one physician.
* Sterilization services are not available locally, and the depot holders are not particularly anxious to motivate the women for this procedure, even when indicated.

Although all conclusions concerning the effectiveness of the Project must be considered tentative until a detailed analysis of the data is available, it is obvious that the programme has been acceptable to all the communities where it has been implemented. At the time of writing, 150 depots have been established and the continuation rates average 70%. It is estimated that the contraceptive prevalence rates in Howrah district will be over 20% at the end of 2 years, and at least 30% by 3 years. Some of the factors to which the achievement of this Project can be attributed are as follows:

* It is simple, easy to implement, and does not require any major capital investment. 'If we have the commodities and the will, we can do it!'
* The programme is built on the goodwill of the villagers, and the entire community is involved right from the planning phase.
* The depot holder is a local person whom the villagers understand, respect and with whom they feel comfortable.
* The income of the depot holder is directly proportional to her efforts, and this acts as a strong incentive.
* The competitive spirit amongst villagers is exploited, and each community tries to outdo the other.
* The Head Office supervises, guides and coordinates the programme, but does not unnecessarily interfere at the village level unless indicated.
* The oral contraceptives are very well accepted and the minor inconvenience of the side-effects far outweigh the burden of pregnancy.
* Constant and abundant availability of contraceptives is always ensured.
* The project is designed to achieve self-sufficiency in 5 years.
* Enlightened donors have significantly contributed to the progress by offering encouragement, allowing flexibility, and not imposing any unnecessary requirements or restrictions.

With a *little* bit of luck, and a *lot* of careful planning, the Howrah CBD Project is rapidly proving to be a great success. It is sincerely hoped that this is just the beginning, and that similar programmes will spring up all over the country to fulfil the unmet needs of India's millions.

Bibliography

Gardner, J. S., Wolff, R. J., Gillespie, D. and Duncan, G. W. (eds.) (1976). *Village and Household Availability of Contraceptives. (Seattle: Battelle)*

Potts, M., Kessel, E. and Bhiwandiwala, P. (1977). *Taking Family Planning to the World's Poor.* (Research Triangle Park: International Fertility Research Program)

Foreit, J. R., Gorosh, M. E., Gillespie, D. G. and Merrit, C. G. (1978). Community-based and commercial contraceptive distribution: an inventory and appraisal. *Population Reports,* J, 19

Potts, D. M. (1976). The implementation of family planning programmes. *Proceedings of the Royal Society of London, B,* **195**, 213

7

Taking family planning to the community – Bombay, India

Datta Pai

DEMOGRAPHIC PROBLEMS	116
THE FAMILY PLANNING PROGRAMME	117
New directions	118
Progress and problems	119
The current plan	120
TAKING STERILIZATION TO THE PEOPLE	121
Railway station surgeries	121
Camp approach	121
Overcoming fears	122
INVOLVEMENT	124
INCENTIVES/DISINCENTIVES	125
UNIFORM LAW	126
Separation from politics	127
THE PRIVATE SECTOR	127
SOLUTIONS	129
Recommended strategy	130
Targets	131
Services	
CONCLUSIONS	132

DEMOGRAPHIC PROBLEMS

Today, the greatest challenge facing mankind is rapid population growth. This problem demands the attention of all nations – east and west, large and small, developed and developing. While the developed countries have successfully overcome this challenge, most of the developing countries have yet to find a solution. In these countries population growth consumes most of the economic gains, condemning people to continued poverty. Too rapid population growth hinders a nation's ability to progress and to satisfy the growing demands of the people for a better life.

India is facing such a critical situation. In spite of achieving remarkable records in planned economic development, the condition of the common man has not improved. Since independence, India has added 250 million people to its population, which is equivalent to the entire population of the USSR, a country six times the area of India. Food production has increased 100%; industrial progress has advanced over 200%. More and more jobs are being created. Still the standard of living of an average Indian has remained more or less unchanged during the last 25 years. Per capita income is about Rs.1000* compared to 6000 dollars in the USA or West Germany, or 4000 dollars in Japan. There is large scale unemployment and destitution in the country, due to tremendous increase in population growth.

The existing population in relation to resources is already large. India, which has 2.5% of the world's area and 1.5% of the world's income, has to support 15% of the world's population – a huge population of 630 millions increasing at the rate of 2% per annum. We are finding it difficult to provide adequate levels of food, clothing, shelter, education, employment and basic amenities to the existing population. On top of this, every year we have to find resources for an additional 13 million people – 125 thousand schools, 400 thousand teachers, 2.5 million houses, 200 million metres of cloth, 2 million tonnes of food grains and 4 million jobs. Put another way, every year India adds to her number the equivalent of the total population of Australia, a country with two and a half times the land area of India.

Discoveries in the field of science and medicine have helped control death rates to an unprecedented extent. By the same token we must also limit the birth rate and family size until the population is stabilized. While death rates have dropped steeply from 48 per thousand at the beginning of this century to 15 per thousand today, birth rates have declined by a smaller proportion from 46 per thousand to only 35 per thousand. The wide gap between the death and birth rates leads to a large increase in the total population. While,

*US$ 1 = 8 rupees

during the first 50 years of the century, the Indian population increased by 100 million, during just one decade between 1961 and 1971 the increase in population reached the staggering figure of 110 millions. The death rate will go down further to 10 per thousand. Unless we bring down the birth rate quickly, the net addition to the population will continue to be large and the economic condition of the people will get worse.

THE FAMILY PLANNING PROGRAMME

India has one of the world's oldest and largest family planning programmes. Long before the Government spelled out its population policy, several social leaders, intellectuals, doctors and some organizations had been campaigning for family limitation. It was this voluntary movement which paved the way for a government-formulated policy. The Planning Commission, which was appointed in 1950, recommended that a programme for family limitation and population control should

* obtain an accurate picture of factors contributing to the rapid population increase in India;
* discover suitable techniques of family planning and devise methods by which knowledge of these techniques could be widely disseminated;
* give advice on family planning as an integral part of service in government and public hospitals.

The small sum of 6.5 million rupees was provided in the first 5 year plan. The emphasis was on research into the physiological and medical aspects of human fertility and also on the various methods of family planning, to determine their suitability, acceptability and effectiveness. Government hospitals and health centres were required to give advice on methods of family planning to married persons who required such advice for reasons of health. At the same time, the rhythm method (safe period) was given a trial and Dr Abraham Stone was invited to offer advice on establishing pilot studies using the rhythm method. The choice of technique was a bad one and although the method had achieved partial success in western countries where the population was educated, in India, due to ignorance amongst women and wide variation in the 'safe period', the method failed. Thus, during the first five year plan period, nothing worthwhile was done towards controlling the population. Even the modest budget allotted was never fully spent.

During the second 5 year plan period a clinical approach was emphasized. The number of service centres increased from 147 to 4167. Research activities were extended to the fields of demography and communication and a voluntary sterilization programme was introduced in many states. The clinical approach was based on the assumption that eligible couples would walk in for advice and service to family planning clinics voluntarily. However, without education and propaganda the response was poor. Therefore, due to lack of direction and involvement at the top level, during the first 10 years after the programme was approved by the government the results were poor.

New directions

In the third plan, the Family Planning Programme did receive some impetus. It had been critically reviewed in 1963 by a special committee and on its recommendation, far-reaching changes were made in the staffing pattern and a new look was given to the programme. The 'extension' approach paved the way for the building up of the programme in subsequent years. If the norm of a small family was to gain voluntary acceptance, the need for education had to acquire a new dimension and force. If services had to be provided, they would have to be available near home, through a close network of public health centres and sub-centres in the rural areas and of hospitals and family welfare centres in urban areas. It was also realized that the actual rate of population growth was increasing at 2% per annum against 1.25% envisaged in the earlier plans. It became clear that specific targets had to take the place of previously vague objectives.

For the first time, a relationship between the reduction in the birth rate and the time element was established. The aim was to lower the birth rate to 25 per thousand by 1976. All the important sectors of the new strategy were strengthened. Education and motivational facilities were increased many times and publicity efforts intensified. Services were made more efficient and extended into more remote areas. Efforts were made to involve community leaders and make family planning a people's movement. A liberal sum of 270 million rupees was allotted for the promotion of the programme. The third plan laid some emphasis on sterilization programmes. An attempt was also made to integrate family planning activities with the maternity and child health (MCH) services, so it would be better accepted by ensuring the health of mothers and longevity of children already born. Integration strengthened the campaign by capitalizing on the skills of workers at every level and by the fact that MCH workers were already accepted by the community. There were greater opportunities in the antenatal, postnatal and paediatric clinics for family planning motivation.

As a result of these progressive steps, there was increased awareness among families of the need for limiting family size and results improved towards the end of the third plan. The unique symbol 'the red triangle' helped create the necessary social climate for controlling the population and wide publicity helped the cause. It made the people conscious of the programme, although the acceptance rate was still low. Incentives and disincentives were officially introduced in some states and the introduction of 'competition' among states and recognition of individual merit added some teeth to the programme. The assurance by the Central Government in Delhi of 100% assistance to the family planning programme (earlier 25% of expenditure was borne by the States) for a period of 10 years prompted the State governments to work with greater enthusiasm. The improvement and strengthening of staff helped the State government to spread the message of family planning to the countryside. The IUD was first introduced as a contraceptive method in August 1966. The free supply of *Nirodh* condoms and their open distribution helped to remove inhibitions. With the large allocation of funds, it was possible to involve more and more institutions and voluntary agencies. Some of the progressive industrialists adopted a liberal policy and gave handsome incentive money to staff accepting family planning. The medical profession also moved into the campaign – although still hesitantly. The voluntary sterilization programme picked up and numbers rose from 100 000 sterilizations performed in 1961 to 400 000 sterilizations in 1965.

Efforts to consolidate the programme organization were intensified during the interplan period (1966–69) and the period was notable for the introduction of the 'camp' approach to voluntary sterilization. Sterilization camps proved an ideal way to take the family planning to the people and the response was tremendous. During the 3 year period (1966–69) over 700 million rupees were spent and 4 million sterilizations were performed.

Progress and problems

The fourth national plan made family planning the kingpin of the plan. Family limitation came to be recognized as an essential and inescapable ingredient of development. A liberal and substantial provision of 3300 million rupees was made for the family planning programme. Mass vasectomy camps, where higher than usual incentives were given, produced encouraging results and during the two years 1971–73 over 5 million voluntary sterilizations were done in India. However, in the last year of the plan, the mass vasectomy camps were discontinued, as a result of some adverse criticism, and there was a drastic reduction in the allotment of funds due to financial stringency. The number of sterilizations dropped to a bare 900 000 in 1973–74. Overall, although the programme did show some impressive records during the fourth plan, the achievements still fell short of the target, which for the fourth plan had been 15 million sterilizations, 6.6 million IUD acceptors and 10 million users of conventional contraceptives: the actual achievement was 10, 2.4 and 4.1 million respectively. The plan had set a goal of protecting a cumulative total of 28 million couples, but reached only 19 million. Better results would have been achieved if sufficient funds had been made available towards the end of the plan and if mass vasectomy camps had been continued.

The current plan

The approach to the fifth plan stresses the objectives of stabilizing the population over a reasonable period as at 'the very centre of planned development'. The total provision made for the family welfare programmes is 5160 million rupees. The targets fixed for the fifth plan are higher for sterilization (18 million), but less for IUDs and conventional contraceptives. Emphasis is placed on sterilizations with a view to lowering the birth rate of 30 per thousand by the end of the plan. During the last 3 years (1974–77) about 12 million sterilizations out of the planned 18 million were performed. Over 8 million were done in 1976–77 – the period of 'Emergency' rule. During this time some cases of 'compulsion' occurred, particularly in the North Indian States. As a result of these excesses, programmes suffered a serious setback. Less than 1 million sterilizations were reported in 1977–78, against 3 million during 1972–73 (Table 1).

TABLE 1 Indian government family planning statistics

	'Emergency' April–Oct 76	*Janata Party April–Oct 77*	*% change*
Vasectomy	2 850 000	63 000	−97
Female sterilization	918 000	284 000	−69
IUDs	257 000	106 000	−58
Other methods	3 291 000	2 700 000	−18
(condom sales)			+25
Abortions	146 000	110 000	−24

In summary, the government programme has been able to deliver large numbers of sterilizations, although it has rarely met its targets and during the Emergency compulsion was used illegally in some areas. The key issue is how to take services to the bulk of the population in an effective, but non-coercive way.

TAKING STERILIZATION TO THE PEOPLE

Maharashtra is one of the most progressive states in India and has been the torch bearer in several social reform movements. In keeping with the tradition, the state and most especially the state capital, Bombay, has been a pioneer in family planning.

Railway station surgeries

In the later 1960s the man seeking a vasectomy was no longer required to attend a hospital – which is traditionally perceived as a dangerous place in India. Instead the choice of male sterilization was brought to the people; simple surgeries were set up on railway stations. Hundreds of thousands of people crowd the mainline terminals in Bombay each day. The operation became less threatening and more available when brought to such a workaday place. The response of the people was dramatic.

In the 10 years before taking vasectomy out of hospitals, 3500 operations had been done. This number was exceeded within a few months of the railway station service. The Indian government was to comment later 'Ten times ten years' performance in ten months in Greater Bombay'.

Camp approach

The camp approach in the vasectomy programme was the singular invention of Maharashtra State and later adopted in other states. The idea is to provide temporary sterilization facilities near colonies, slum areas and villages. It is the best way to take the programme to the people, as it permits deployment of motivational and medical expertise in situations where it is ordinarily unavailable. The combination of motivation and action in camps helped Maharashtra to win many national awards in family planning.

The 'continuing camps' in crowded railway stations have just been noted. Additionally, four mobile family planning operation theatres were set up in covered old buses to take vasectomy services to factory premises, markets, slums and other places where people gather together. Mobile booths, made of bamboos and banners, have been the recent culmination of the camp approach – tentacles triggering family planning action in communities and neighbourhoods of Greater Bombay.

Overcoming fears

Tradition and illiteracy are recognized impediments in engineering any social change. But, the greatest hurdle in family planning is fear. Fears, anxieties, apprehensions and suspicions are built into every human.

Fear of insecurity: the tradition of having many children has deep roots in the human past, when the family unit was the only insurance against improvidence; death was common and life a struggle for survival. High infant mortality rates and death rates induced a desire for more children as a reaction to insecurity. Present-day talk of decreasing death rates cannot easily overcome such traditional concepts from the past, nor are they convincing in communities where infant mortality rates continue to be higher than 100 per 1000 live births, as in some developing countries. Moreover, poorly developed social security measures do not engender the necessary confidence to accept a small family norm. Under the circumstances, family planning as a programme of family welfare can be meaningful only through improved survival. Though the government of India initiated activities through family welfare and planning centres, the welfare component could not be developed in a commensurate manner, because of evident difficulties in terms of funds, staff and facilities. Some experts infer that the stated integrated approach lacked the necessary commitment. Whichever may be the reason, mass acceptance of family planning will be determined by ensuring improved survival of children. Most of the surveys organized in Greater Bombay have indicated that couples do not accept family planning unless they have two children, one of whom is a son. Many do not accept sterilization unless they have two sons, irrespective of religion. If sterilization is considered as a method of choice, increasing security through survival should be built into the family planning programme.

Fear of body injury: another frequent fear which explains the existing disparity in knowledge and practice of family planning is triggered by problems of safety. No method is one hundred per cent safe and the occasional complication provides a factual basis for dissemination of rumours. Unfortunately, lack of follow-up led to the collapse of the IUD programmes in India in the 1960s. Vasectomy and tubectomy programmes are plodding a stereotyped path of rise and fall because of inadequate vigilance in ensuring the quality and continuity of aftercare. The safety of a method lies in its effective demonstration. The Greater Bombay experiment in vasectomy has been one such effective demonstration.

There was a method in the madness of railway station vasectomy. Fear of body injury associated with operations and hospitals was overcome by instituting the first hygienic operations at railway stations. This simple step changed the psychology of the people. The necessary vigilance was exercised to reduce the complications to a minimum and to mobilize the necessary curative resources if and when complications occurred. Thus vasectomy was proved to be a safe, simple operation in the eyes of the people. In a city where only one vasectomy used to be performed each day, the programme spiralled up to an average of 200 sterilizations per day and the tempo has been maintained throughout.

Fear of sex injury: sex is a deep-rooted driving force. Fear of sex injury dissuades many men from contraception. (Complications of hirsutism in females using oral contraception led to non-acceptance during the earlier period.) Sex dissatisfaction is the major drawback of the condom. Fear of possible impotence has threatened the progress of the vasectomy programme. A recent study conducted in Greater Bombay indicated that about 3% of individuals indicate an improvement in sex relations after vasectomy, mainly due to the removal of the fear of pregnancy. However, about 5% complain of diminution of libido. In a large majority of these cases, evidence of poor motivation and /or improper treatment of complications led to dissatisfaction and rejection. Under the circumstances, increased inputs in motivational and follow-up support of the programme are required in overcoming the fear of sex injury.

Fear of family injury: the message 'two or three children are enough' is interpreted by an individual through his own life experiences. To him death is an ever present risk. As already stated, one of the barriers to the acceptance of sterilization is the fear of death of the children or the spouse, as sterilization is considered as a drastic irreversible method. The greater challenge, therefore, in the mass movement for voluntary sterilization is the mobilization of total resources to make recanalization a greater reality. Of the 615 000 sterilized individuals in Greater Bombay, only 698 individuals sought recanalization. The need is not great but the confidence it generates will accelerate the pace of acceptance.

Fear of moral injury: everyone is a moralist to a greater or lesser extent. Fears of body injury, sex injury and family injury can be overcome through a scientific approach. Fear of moral injury has roots in philosophy and ethics and is a formidable handicap against family planning. People argue that family planning will lead to promiscuous sex indulgence – a permissive society. It may undermine the moral fibre of future generations. The man who worries over a bachelor taking condoms may not agree with the philosophy of preventing unwanted children. He may not agree that immoral people are sufficiently motivated to get the necessary implements through other channels. He may not agree that the greatest moral sin is to punish innocence by begetting an unwanted child, who cannot complain, into a home of chronic want and misery. Moralists die hard. Unfortunately, morality is woven around sex. In its extremist form, it is manifested in the shape of religious objection. In Greater Bombay, an effort is made to break down the morality, secrecy and shyness around sex by instituting information-cum-condom distribution centres at all railway stations and through other channels of mass communication. Increase in condom use from 90 to 35 000 per day is only incidental. As a triggering mechanism, it is ushering in an insidious but constructive change.

Fear of group injury: the greatest iceberg in the path of family planning is differential acceptance by various religions, regional and socio-economic groups. Unfortunately, target-orientated family planning programmes have occasionally become programmes of convenience, rather than programmes of conviction. Willing families accept fertility limitation and the resistant continue to breed. Unless greater efforts are made in areas of higher resistance, the programme will not attain a representative character and this may ultimately undermine its future progress.

INVOLVEMENT

To make the family planning programme a peoples' programme, it is necessary to involve all sections of the community. In a democracy, government machinery alone can never achieve meaningful success unless individuals and institutions are totally involved. One of the distinctive features of the Maharashtra programme has been the complete involvement of *Zilla Parishads* (district organizations). Since *Zilla Parishads* are run by local leaders, the implementation of welfare schemes, like family planning, becomes more effective as they can influence people from within their respective localities. Total involvement of leaders in rural areas has greatly contributed to the success of the family planning movement in rural sectors in Maharashtra.

In the Greater Bombay programme, heavy emphasis is placed on involvement of all sections of the population, including leaders of the community, representatives of institutions and industries and medical practitioners. The help of voluntary organizations is sought. These include community associations and institutions like womens' organizations, tenants' associations and service organizations like the Lions, Rotary and Jaycees. Elected representatives are also being approached to give the programme a push. The assistance of teachers, lawyers, journalists and students is gratefully accepted.

A big effort has been made to involve the 5000 medical practitioners from the city in the campaign. Practising doctors are among the best motivators, because the family doctor is usually treated with respect by the patients. If the need of the small family norm is explained by the family doctor to his patients, the chances of family planning acceptance are improved. To enable the medical practitioners to do a proper job, one day orientation and involvement programmes have been organized. Here, doctors are apprised of the latest methods of contraception and advised as regards techniques of motivation.

INCENTIVES/DISINCENTIVES

Incentives/disincentives have played a major role in the promotion of the programme. Higher incentives have always brought better results. The Indian family planning programme, by and large, has been a voluntary programme and an effort is made to motivate people for family planning by education and persuasion. Education takes time and hence the need for other methods and strategies for involving greater numbers of people. Cash incentives are a supplementary measure to hasten the process of adoption of family planning. A cash incentive need not be considered as a bribe. It is rather in the nature of a 'compensation' for out-of-pocket expenditure and wage loss during the post-operative period. The rationale of the idea is fully justifiable. The 'Small Family Norm Committee' of the government of India states:

'. . . compensation is for meeting out-of-pocket expenses and is not an incentive as such . . . in the long run the real incentive should be the benefit accruing by the practice of small family norm.'

The committee draws attention to the fact that fertility control can be achieved not merely by the dispensation of family planning methods, but also by socioeconomic measures. Their policy, in fact, goes a step further and calls for withdrawal of concessions from those who have more than three children after the declaration of the policy. The committee says:

'Though group acceptance of small family norm can be achieved through mass communication and extension education techniques, incentives and disincentives are essential to trigger off action. Studies have shown a fairly wide gulf between acceptance and practice of family planning. Incentives and disincentives bridge this gulf and lead to positive action.'

The committee even recommends some rebate in life insurance premiums to those who have undergone sterilization after two or three children. It also recommends that the Life Insurance Corporation of India and the Postal Life Insurance should be asked to initiate policies with special benefits redeemable after 18 years of marriage if the family size is restricted to two or three children. National service bonds redeemable after 15 to 20 years may be issued to acceptors of family planning and loans may also be given against these bonds for family projects in rural areas which may have the effect of promoting security to the whole family, especially the parents.

Incentives, then, are designed to encourage and prod an individual to overcome his inhibition or inherited attitudes. Disincentives are the other side of the coin to deter him from plunging headlong into a family neither he nor the country can afford. An incentive scheme can be three-tiered. The scheme can be individual, family or community-based. In the case of individual and family based schemes, it is sometimes argued that the danger of misuse is inherent. An individual may succumb to the temptation of immediate monetary gain and make an inappropriate choice. Such a possibility, even if remote, can be pre-empted through community-based incentive schemes. Since the entire scheme is community-based, a successful outcome generates popular enthusiasm and participation. The size of the community to which the incentive scheme is to be extended can be anything between 2000 and 6000 individuals. Inevitably, the programme gains a new dimension; what is good for the individual is also good for the community and what is necessary for the community as a whole is good for an individual member.

Incentives, when introduced along with disincentives, become more effective. Disincentives do not mean denial of any right, but withdrawal of concessions in the interest of the society. The government of Maharashtra had taken certain steps to withdraw some concessions prior to the new population policy in 1977. These concessions included grant of loans, subsidies, free medical facilities, maternity benefits, allotment of quarters to government servants, allotment of tenements in the State Housing Board Colonies. Those who do not restrict the size of the family to three living children were to be denied these concessions.

UNIFORM LAW

Recently, discussions have taken place regarding proposals to legislate for a small family. The President has suggested that if different political parties could discuss and come to an agreement, legislation could be put through to limit family size. The law could provide for some sort of penalty or disincentive to those with more than, say, 3 or 4 children. The law once passed would apply uniformly to all states and all communities.

Legislation to limit the family is not a new idea in India. During 1976 the States of Maharashtra, Haryana and Punjab all passed legislation for compulsory sterilization after a specified number of children. Although these laws were passed by the state assemblies with large majorities, it was thought at the federal level that these bills were too drastic. In any case. these were to be enforced only in three states. What is contemplated now is a uniform law to be applicable to all states.

Instead of sterilization alone, persons could adopt any method of family planning to control the family. Such a law could induce people who already have three or four children, but who are not taking any definite step to limit the family, to take some positive action. It is likely that a bill of this type could secure a wide measure of public support if adequately discussed in public. A law, or laws of this type, eventually might be applicable to all countries for bringing uniform action to tackle a major problem confronting mankind.

Separation from politics

Population control is a national welfare which promotes the interests of all sections of the people, strengthening the economic and social structure of the country. As such, it is desirable that all political parties wholeheartedly work for the propagation of the programme. If the party in power takes reasonable and legitimate steps to advance the cause of family planning, all parties should lend support to such measures rather than oppose them merely to gain short-term political advantage. Politics should be completely separated from welfare programmes. There should be a national commitment to a population control programme. If possible, programmes should be planned, implemented and evaluated by an autonomous body consisting of professionals (medical and social scientists, demographers, communication and management experts and others) who enjoy the confidence of the country.

THE PRIVATE SECTOR

Bombay established the first family planning hospital in 1971, as a centralized specialist institution where total family planning services including treatment of sterilization complications and recanalization of sterilization operations were made available with the greatest care. This ultimately led to a private popular model at Pearl Centre where free family planning services, abortion at normal cost and subsidized medical care (Table 2) are made available on a low profit basis. The Pearl Centre achieves high turnover through a daring communications system and demonstrates the potential for quality effort in voluntary family planning action. It can be the model for an extended network of non-governmental action.

TABLE 2 User charges at charitable clinic (Pearl Centre, Bombay)

Procedure	*Rupee*	*$US*
Abortion	70	9
Delivery	70	9
Delivery (and 1 week clinic stay)	200	25
Pregnancy test	15	2
Non-family planning consultation	20	3
Sterilization and IUD insertion	free	

TABLE 3 Utilization of private charitable clinic (Pearl Centre, Bombay)

Procedure		*Year*	
	1974–75	*1975–76*	*1976–77*
Abortions	3227	6101	8611
Sterilizations	447	3196	2002
Oral contraceptive users	—	1763	2680
IUD insertions	181	586	534

The facility occupies 370 square metres, has three operation theatres and 25 beds. There is one full-time resident doctor and four part-time physicians and a full-time non-medical manager. Salaries include incentives and profit sharing. It is estimated that the clinic has performed nearly one third of the legal abortions done in Bombay, complications are low and there is an 80% follow-up (Table 3).

SOLUTIONS

Most of the governments in the developing world have realized the seriousness of the problem and embarked on population control programmes. However, the success in achieving substantial reduction in population growth has been limited. Due to government propaganda through mass media and through the efforts of various voluntary agencies, the peoples' awareness of the population problem is widespread, but often the number of people who actually practise family planning remains severely limited. The problem is to bridge the gap between awareness and acceptance as early as possible, with minimum inputs. Established attitudes and values may have to be changed. The tremendous task of changing a whole people's attitude calls for innovation and technical skill of a high order and requires dedicated, full-time effort by medical practitioners, auxiliaries, social workers and field workers.

Studies indicate that human fertility rarely declines unless certain basic social needs are satisfied. Birth rates drop in response to reduced infant mortality and improved child survival. Hence, emphasis has to be laid on maternal and child health services, including antenatal, perinatal and postnatal care, nutrition and immunization. Current thinking is to make family planning services as comprehensive and broad-based as possible – the philosophy of total health and well-being of the family which alone can make parents realize that a small family is in their own interest. There has been a move to link family planning with development and welfare measures, such as the provision of drinking water and electricity in the villages, food supply, literacy and good medical care. While it may be ideal to make services broad-based, it should be borne in mind that with limited funds available, it may not be possible to pursue all these welfare items at the same time. There is a danger that while tackling multifarious welfare programmes, the family planning programme may drop into the background. For instance, in a country like India, where 50% of the population is below poverty level, the mere supply of food could take up all the money allotted for health and welfare services. It is necessary, therefore, to give priority to maternal and child health programmes, minimum medical care and family planning. Funds allotted for family planning easily get diverted into non-family planning areas. Workers like to devote their time to easier, popular items, like the distribution of vitamin tablets, immunization – providing health care but neglecting family planning.

Recommended strategy

The present objective in India is to reduce the birth rate by one point per thousand per year over the next ten years, so that the birth rate reaches 25/1000 by 1984 at the end of the 6th plan. This goal calls for a gargantuan effort. So far, over 27 million sterilizations, 6 million IUD insertions and 4 million users of conventional contraceptives have been achieved. At present only 25% of 115 million couples in the reproductive age group are protected. Forty five per cent require protection in order to reduce the birth rate to 25/1000. In real terms this requires the sterilization of at least 3.5 million couples every year till 1984, apart from 1 million IUD insertions and 5 million new users of conventional methods. Nearly 3 million sterilizations were done in 1975–76 (during 1976–77 the total number of sterilizations was over 8 million) but this was an exceptionally good performance. It is not easy to repeat this achievement. The present atmosphere is not conducive to acceleration of the sterilization programme. The possibility of reducing the birth rate to 25 per thousand by 1984 looks remote, unless successful ideas and actions are replicated with confidence.

A plan of action to cover the total population (with minimum loss of time) with family planning services is needed as a part of an integrated package of health, family planning, nutrition and maternal and child health services at all levels. The peripheral unit of family planning action in India should be a sub-centre with an approximate population of 5000, entrusted to a multipurpose (family planning) worker (MFW) who would be responsible for the organization of family planning, consisting of:

Survey: to identify couples and needs. In a unit of 5000 in India the average family will have five members and there will be 1000 couples. One hundred couples (10%) are likely to be subfertile; 450 couples (45%) have three or less living children; 450 couples (45%) have four or more living children and therefore are definitely eligible only for sterilization. A few couples with 2 or 3 living children from the earlier group are also likely to accept sterilization.

A family planning worker must cover 20 couples a day and will therefore complete her round every 2 months – not more than every 3 months under any circumstances. She must prepare an eligible couple register (identification number; name of husband and wife, ages of couple; number of living boys and living girls; method currently used; advice given). Additional information on health and nutrition may also be recorded if relevant.

Motivation: this means reaching the minds of the people to bring about the desired attitude change – to give simple and meaningful information about the why and how of family planning; to identify and overcome anxieties, apprehension, suspicions and fears (see section on overcoming fears); to increase awareness, knowledge and conviction; and, finally, to precipitate action. Motivation is as important as medical expertise in the implementation of family planning programmes. Hence, some of the routine measures that must be practised at unit and *taluka* level are outlined below.

- An individual family approach to eligible couples. This method can have great influence on the individual. Barriers that an individual may perceive in the way of adopting a new practice can be removed, misinformation can be corrected and negative attitudes reversed through this approach.
- Small group meetings can be organized which supplement individual approaches and provide for interaction among more people. It is useful if one or two satisfied adopters participate in such meetings.
- Formal and informal village leaders have a crucial role to play in the promotion of family planning programmes and should be located and trained.
- It has been observed that satisfied adopters remain passive while those that experience any complication broadcast their negative experiences. The MFW should develop a plan to identify satisfied adopters and encourage them to communicate their satisfaction to potential users in their own peer groups. In rural areas, a potential user may be influenced to a greater extent by a peer group member who is a satisfied adopter than any other communicator.
- Village *dais* (traditional birth attendants) and indigenous medical practitioners can be useful allies when they talk about family planning to their clients. Before they are requested to do so, information sessions should be arranged for them, so that their doubts about the advantages of the various methods may be removed.

Targets

The minimum motivation targets for all family planning workers shall be 8 group meetings and 8 successful equivalent sterilizations (ES*) every month.

---

*ES = equivalent sterilization is two abortions, two oral Pill users, three loops or ten conventional contraceptive users.

This means that every sub-centre will achieve nearly 100 ES per year or 20 ES per 1000 population per year in keeping with short term goals. Fifty sterilizations, either male or female must be achieved every year by every MFW.

Services

The MFW should supply conventional contraceptives and oral Pills during her rounds. A three months' supply should be issued routinely. Clients requiring medical expertise (including menstrual regulation) should be referred to appropriately staffed centres according to a fixed schedule. A mini-camp should be held once every year in the sub-centres for operative procedures (for IUD, vasectomy and female sterilization). The day for the mini-camp should be decided early in the year so that a family planning campaign would lead up to the camp.

Follow-up has often been the weakest link in the chain of family planning action. To give adequate emotional and therapeutic support to the client, the MFW must arrange follow-up visits to anyone adopting a family planning method before the end of the week, before the end of the month, once every three months, and thereafter to ensure total satisfaction of the client and treat complications, if any, very speedily.

CONCLUSIONS

The key to successful family planning lies as much in terms of human commitment as it does in the techniques provided. A sub-centre family planning programme implementation committee should be convened by the MFW as early as possible, which may consist of a resident member of the union; one member from any of the developmental agencies; any other important individual; a medical practitioner; a representative each of an educational institution and an industrial organization and any other person who may be useful. Family planning workers and the community must generate the necessary conviction and involvement to transform the programme into a mass movement.

Bibliography

Bhatt, R. V., Pachauri, S., Pathak, N. D. and Chauhan, L. (1978). Female sterilization in small camp settings in rural India. *Studies in Family Planning,* **9** (2), 39

Chandrasekhar, S. (1970). *India's Population.* (Meerut: Meenakshi Prakashan)
Krishnakumar, S. (1972). Kerala's pioneering experiment in massive vasectomy camps. *Studies in Family Planning,* **3** (8), 177
Mahmood Mamdani (1972). *The Myth of Population Control.* (New York: Monthly Review Press)
Mehta, P. V. and Pathak, K. B. (1977). Some problems of compulsion in family planning. *Journal of Biosocial Science,* **9,** 273
Potts, M. (1970). BMT 2118. *Family Planning,* **19** (2), 43
Wyon, J. B. and Gordon, J. E. (1971). *The Khanna Study.* (Cambridge, Mass.: Harvard University Press)

8

Social marketing – Sri Lanka and Bangladesh

Terry Louis
and
Robert Ciszewski

COMMERCIAL MARKETING – AN ADAPTATION 136

SRI LANKA: THE FIRST NATIONWIDE APPLICATION OF SOCIAL MARKETING 137

FORMULATING TARGETS 138

IMPLEMENTATION 138

SRI LANKA: PERFORMANCE 139

SRI LANKA: EVALUATION 142
Cost-effectiveness 143
Rapid feedback and flexibility of management 145

SRI LANKA: CONCLUSIONS 146

BANGLADESH: EXPANDED APPLICATION OF SOCIAL MARKETING 147

BARRIERS 147

PROMOTION 148

AVAILABILITY AND ACCEPTABILITY 148

BANGLADESH: PERFORMANCE 149
Cost-effectiveness 149
Towards self-sufficiency 150

CONCLUSIONS 150

COMMERCIAL MARKETING – AN ADAPTATION

Population Services International (PSI), a charitable organization, was commissioned in 1973 by the International Planned Parenthood Federation (IPPF) to initiate a contraceptive marketing programme in Sri Lanka. At first, the management was entirely in the hands of PSI and IPPF provided funds to cover promotional and administrative costs and a free supply of contraceptives, which were imported without tax into the country.

The goal of the programme was to demonstrate (1) that commercial marketing techniques could significantly increase the number of couples using reliable, modern contraceptives, and (2) that unit costs would be as low as or lower than those of clinic-based programmes.

The pragmatic relationship between a product's attributes and the consumer's needs is the backbone of all commercial marketing. In the context of family planning, 'the marketing task is to influence the choice process through actions that seek to increase the attractiveness and accessibility of the fertility control product'. Family planning programme developers have experimented with non-profit versions of commercial models as alternatives to the more common clinic models. The use of marketing techniques for the advancement of family planning and other social programmes has been called 'social marketing' by Kotler and Zaltman (1971).

A review of the literature on social marketing programmes in India, Indonesia and Kenya suggests that although its impact on fertility may be difficult to assess, the commercial orientation offers several advantages. It appears that programmes mounted along commercial lines have the following advantages:

* They can be created rapidly;
* They can harness established channels of distribution and require very little capital expenditure;
* The monetary incentives built into the distribution chain can provide for rapid programme growth while reducing service costs;
* Small professional marketing management teams can provide the necessary professional management and give the required expertise and flexibility to the decision-making process;
* Orientation of a contraceptive programme towards consumers usually results in large increases in awareness of the product among potential acceptors.

'Marketing is a consumer orientated philosophy of business. In its simplest form the philosophy is that the consumer is the most important person, and therefore the objective is to first identify the wants of the consumers and then to bring together and transform men, materials and money into goods and services that will satisfy these wants; and then perform all the functions that will enable the consumer to voluntarily part with his money, and to take in exchange goods and services that satisfy his wants.' If this philosophy is to be accepted, then it is necessary to consciously and consistently use a series of inter-related methods and techniques to ensure that the activities are in accordance with the philosophy of marketing. The inter-related techniques and methods are commonly called the individual activities that constitute the marketing mix, or the individual parts of the marketing function. Social marketing does not vary or differ in philosophy from consumer marketing. The only change in the mix is that the activity is directed for a social benefit and not necessarily profit. The correct marketing mix will have the right product, at the right price, in the right package, with the right distribution, right advertising and right management of the product and distribution.

SRI LANKA: THE FIRST NATIONWIDE APPLICATION OF SOCIAL MARKETING

The first task of PSI management in Sri Lanka was to identify the wants of the consumer in terms of family planning in order to offer the *right product*. Here *market research* played an important part. The function of market research is to deliver the information necessary with which one can identify consumer wants. The research carried out on the knowledge, acceptance and practice (KAP) of family planning provided the following conclusions:

* family planning was already a well-known concept in Sri Lanka;
* there was a reasonable degree of knowledge about contraception;
* a high degree of approval of the need for family planning existed;
* there was a genuine intention to space and to restrict family size;
* there was a significant willingness to use contraceptive methods;
* the degree of family planning practice was low.

The main reasons for approving family planning were:

* the belief that spacing children provides better health for both mother and child;
* spacing children confers economic benefits.

It was concluded that there was a marketing opportunity and this led to the strategy to market the condom as a product acceptable to the consumer. The objective was to persuade a significant number of married couples to fulfil the need for family planning through condom acceptance and use.

FORMULATING TARGETS

In keeping with the marketing model, targets were formulated in marketing terms and then transformed into demographic terms. The first-year target (Table 1) was set at 1% of the estimated adult males with a discretionary cash income. Since there were no available use-rate data for condom acceptors in Sri Lanka, the sales target for the first year was based upon the government of India's estimate that '72 condoms are enough to protect one user for one year'. At that rate, 28 000 couples (1.6% of married women of reproductive age) would require two million condoms per year. A revised estimate of the actual use rate for Sri Lanka was ascertained by surveying *Preethi* acceptors one year after the programme was launched.

TABLE 1 First-year social marketing targets (Sri Lanka, 1973–74)

Item	*Number*
Total population (1972 estimate)	13 200 000
Estimated number of adult males with disposable cash income (21%)	2 800 000
First-year target (1%)	28 000

IMPLEMENTATION

The condom marketing programme began in May 1973. During the first six months, a two-person PSI management team assisted by a part-time Sri Lankan consultant, designed the operational plan and commissioned market studies, distribution, advertising and printing by local social agencies and private companies. On 1 October 1973 the programme was launched; during the following 18 months it was monitored, modified, and evaluated under PSI management.

An essential aspect of the programme was the harnessing of an existing nationwide network of retailers to make condoms available to the greatest number of fertile couples in the shortest possible time. Reckitt and Colman (Ceylon) Ltd. – an established and successful marketer of various household products – was commissioned to package and distribute the imported product to its 4000 prime retailers.

A series of consumer preference tests established the various product attributes that would be emphasized in the advertising and education campaigns; this included the brand name *Preethi* (meaning joy and happiness), the package design, and symbol, the launch-period advertising theme, and the price of 40 Sri Lankan cents (US $0.04) for a package of condoms. (Each package contained three foil-wrapped, nipple-ended, lubricated Durex Gossamer condoms, manufactured in England.)

For one month prior to the nationwide launch, *Preethi*'s acceptability to retailers was tested empirically by offering the product and advertising to 200 prime retailers in a rural area; 75% of the retailers readily purchased and displayed a full dispenser of *Preethi* (40 packs of 3 condoms each). A metal sign was displayed outside each shop identifying it as a supplier of *Preethi.* Meanwhile, each of the 4000 prime retailers throughout the nation was given an orientation folder and a sample of *Preethi,* informing him of the product, its functions and benefits. He was also informed that he could purchase stocks the following month, while nationwide advertising was beginning.

On 1 October 1973, nationwide distribution and mass media advertising were initiated. The launch period was designated as two years, which is the time required for a new product in Sri Lanka to settle into the distribution pipeline, be accepted by target retailers, receive any marketing modifications, and find its prime market segment.

SRI LANKA: PERFORMANCE

By 31 March 1975, 18 months after the launch period began, nearly 5.9 million condoms had been distributed, including 5.6 million sold to more than 4000 retailers; 114 000 sold by mail order; and 124 000 given away as free samples. Figure 1 illustrates the dominant role of the retail sector in the first distribution pattern. The higher-than-average volume of sales in the first month is typical of all new products, while data for following months indicate actual replenishment of stocks sold to consumers, plus a slow and steady increase in the number of *Preethi* shops. Mail-order sales began in January 1974; almost 2% of the sales between October 1973 and the end of March 1975 were through the mail. The number of *Preethis* actually used in the 18-month period was estimated to be about 4.9 million (Table 2).

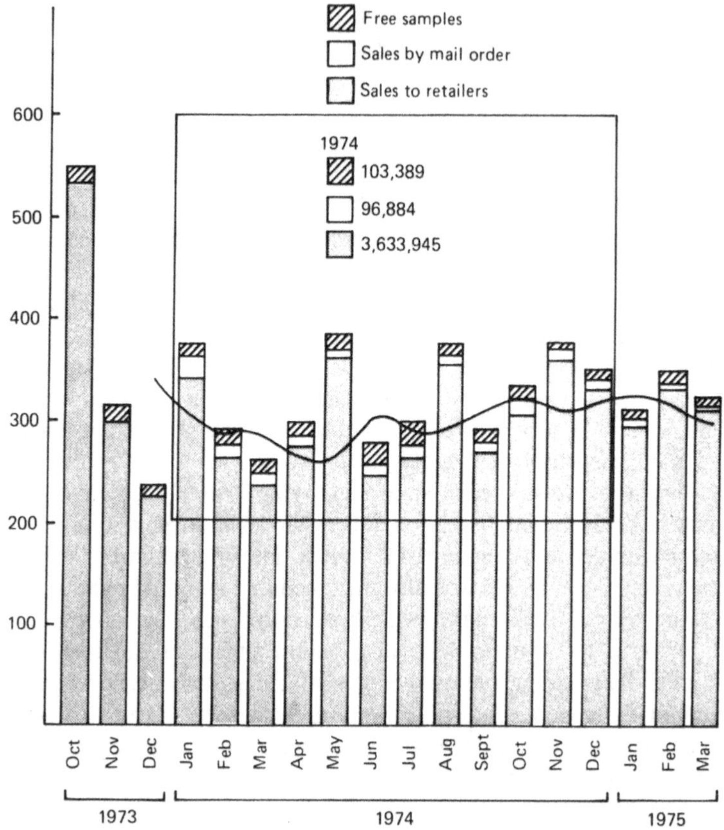

Figure 1 Condom sales in Sri Lanka: 1973–75

The KAP replication surveys indicated that 13% of urban couples and 12% of rural couples were currently using condoms, and that two-thirds of them were using *Preethi*. Thus, an estimated 144 000 couples (8% of 1.8 million married women of reproductive age) were using *Preethi*, with a reported use ranging from 1 to 12 condoms per month, and a computed mean and median use of 62 per year. Acceptors who could not say how many they used were excluded from this calculation.

Results from the KAP survey can be compared with those from a pilot survey of 72% *Preethi* purchasers in 29 randomly chosen urban chemist shops. (Twenty-one additional interviews were discontinued due to the respondents' reported lack of time.) Of the respondents completing interviews, 70% were men aged 25–39; 4% were women; 50% had been married for two

TABLE 2 Condoms *(Preethi)* distributed in first 18 months of programme (October 1973–March 1975)

Item	*Number (thousands)*
Sold to retailers during the first 18 months	5637
Less retailers' inventory*	−738
Total purchased from retailers	4899
Plus mail-order purchases	+114
Total purchased by consumers	5013
Plus samples given to consumers	+124
Total distributed to consumers	5137
Less number unused by consumers	−272
Total used	**4865**

* The retailers' estimated inventory was extrapolated from the physical count of *Preethi* stock-on-hand in a 10% probability sample of *Preethi* retailers. The unused consumers' stocks may be overestimated, since they represent an average of almost two-thirds of a *Preethi* package on hand per acceptor.

to ten years; and 64% had three or less children; 74% had some secondary education, and 46% reported spouses with a similar level of education. All the men reported some degree of employment.

But since only urban chemist shops were sampled in this pilot survey, it is not surprising that high employment and education levels were reported. Future surveys of additional retail strata, particularly rural provisioners' shops, will tend to balance the profile.

Seventy-nine per cent of purchasers lived close to the sampled shop. Ten per cent were making a first purchase and 69% bought one packet of *Preethi* at a time. The mean coital frequency was 10.5 per month and the mean use rate 8.4 condoms per month. However, coital rates and use rates for the sample may be expected to be above average as the sampling design tended to select the most frequent purchasers (and users). Fifty per cent reported using *Preethi* with every coitus, while another 26% said they alternated it with the rhythm method – using *Preethi* during the unsafe part of the cycle. Nineteen per cent of couples had tried oral contraceptives but had discontinued use. Among the 83% who said they would continue with *Preethi,* the three reasons most often given were convenience, dependability and the absence of side effects.

The initial KAP survey was repeated once *Preethi* had been on the market for some time. The results indicated a generally increased awareness of the condom as a family planning method and a high level of knowledge about

Preethi. All those interviewed indicated a greater awareness of *Preethi* than of condoms *per se,* underlining the importance of choosing the right brand name. Most of those who were aware of *Preethi* could describe it correctly. Interestingly, women registered greater knowledge of *Preethi* as a product than knowledge of specific advertising, indicating the transmission of knowledge by interpersonal communication which must have followed on the awareness created in others by the mass media advertising.

SRI LANKA: EVALUATION

'Acceptor' may not be an appropriate word for commercially orientated programmes since it connotes passiveness in the acceptance. It is used here, however, following standard practice. In a commercially orientated programme, the user nearly always purchases the contraceptive, thus playing an active and dynamic role rather than a passive part in the process. 'Acceptor' therefore is used interchangeably with consumer, client, purchaser, and user, while it is understood that in a few cases the acceptor or purchaser may not actually be the user.

Because social marketing programmes are orientated toward serving the consumer's needs by supplying a product, the collection of information on the acceptor at the time of first acceptance, which is intrinsic to clinic procedures, is omitted. Therefore, contraceptive social marketing programmes may be more difficult to evaluate than clinic programmes. To a significant degree, however, survey data can be used to interpret marketing results and to produce measures of impact comparable in utility to those usually generated by clinic programmes. The level of impact can then be compared to input costs to provide indicators of efficiency.

Generally speaking, social marketing programmes produce good input and output data. Costs are readily ascertainable, since programmes are discrete and most of the costs are wholly applied to producing tangible results. Output (sales of contraceptives) are measured routinely each month in terms of sales to retailers, adjusted by the technique of shop auditing to reflect actual customer purchases. This is a simple process compared with the task of assessing the efficiency of clinic-based programmes – particularly those that share facilities and personnel with activities other than family planning, or those that offer various family planning services in addition to contraceptives. Furthermore, clinic-based programmes must contend with the problem of measuring the real use of contraceptive supplies which are distributed free of charge, while in a social marketing programme where people pay for contraceptives, wastage is likely to be slight – especially in a developing country where most people are poor.

Cost-effectiveness

Cost-effectiveness can be determined easily for several aspects of the *Preethi* programme, particularly at the output level. It is most appropriately measured for one calendar year of activity and 1974 has been chosen since it excludes the abnormally high 'selling-in' activity during the first launch months and represents a fairly stable period of consumer purchases (see Figure 1). Costs were higher for 1974 than for later in the programme due to heavy launching inputs, advertising and survey costs. Therefore dollar costs are higher than those anticipated for a more mature programme.

As shown in Tables 3 and 4 over three million condoms were distributed at a net cost of $311 000. Assuming an average use of 72 condoms per couple per year, as the post-launch KAP survey indicated, then *Preethi* provided the equivalent of about 50 000 couple-years of contraception in 1974, at a cost of $6.19 per couple-year, including an advertising cost of $1.76. The cost for each of the 144 000 new acceptors was $2.16, including an advertising cost of $0.62. There was a cost of $0.09 for advertising and instruction for each couple of reproductive age who learned that *Preethi* was a contraceptive used by men (Table 5).

TABLE 3 Estimate of condoms *(Preethi)* distributed in 1974

Item	*Number (thousands)*
Sold to retailers during first 15 months	4705
Less retailers' inventory	−717
Total purchased from retailers	3988
Average purchases for one year (3988 × 12/15)	3191
Plus mail-order purchases	+97
Total purchases by consumers	3288
Plus samples given to consumers	+103
Total received by consumers	3391
Less number unused by consumers	−272
Total used in 1974	**3119**

TABLE 4 Condom *(Preethi)* programme costs in 1974

Item	*Cost (in $US)*
Condoms (at $3.15 per gross)	83 900
Salaries and consultants	43 800
Office expenses and travel	21 800
Surveys	12 900
Advertising and education*	88 600
Mail order and packaging †	29 300
Indirect international costs ‡	50 100
Subtotal	330 400
Less net sales (returned to programme)	19 200
Net cost	**311 200**

Note: All known costs are shown, including shipping, vehicle and equipment depreciation, international travel, evaluation, and PSI head office administration costs. The cost of condoms represents an estimated average for purchases over a period of time.
*Mail order advertising costs are included.
† Mail order postage and packaging costs are included.
‡ Overhead costs such as PSI head-office time and communication costs.

TABLE 5 Summary of the cost-effectiveness of the Sri Lankan condom *(Preethi)* programme in 1974

Measurement	*Calculation*	*Cost in $US*
Net programme cost		
Per capita	311 200÷13 400 000=	0.02
Per acceptor	311 200÷144 000 =	2.16
Per couple-year of contraception	311 200÷50 305 =	6.19
Per total births averted	311 200÷10 000 =	31 00
Per net births averted	311 200÷6 00 =	48.00
Advertising cost		
Per knowledgeable couple	88 600÷960 000 =	0.09
Per acceptor	88 600÷144 000 =	0.62
Per couple-year of contraception	88 600÷50 305 =	1.76

The above analysis of the results and effects of *Preethi* over a short span of time brings to light several strengths and weaknesses of the social marketing model. These need to be examined as they apply to the continuation of the *Preethi* programme in Sri Lanka and to more generalized uses of the model in other countries.

Rapid feedback and flexibility of management

Feedback to management from the field can be obtained very quickly in the marketing model. One example from the distribution chain and one from the advertising programme will illustrate the ease with which modifications can be made.

Improving the retailer's role – Preethi produced an increase in the number of private-sector family planning contact points from 300 to over 4000 in one year. An *ad hoc* survey of a sample of these retailers showed good display of the product, but considerable diffidence in retailers' attitudes toward recommending the use of *Preethi.* Because of their reluctance to recommend the product a 'congratulation kit' was assembled and hand-delivered to each retailer 6 weeks after the survey was made. The kit contained a letter certifying the role of the retailer as a family planner, a preview of forthcoming advertising, and leaflets to be distributed to potential customers. Future surveys of retailers will be needed to ascertain the degree to which these inputs dispelled retailers' shyness about the topic of contraception.

Fine-tuning communications – An excellent response to the first few advertisements offering information and samples led to the development of a full-scale mail-order business. Promotional funds were deployed to produce a variety of advertisements in different media and these brought in more than 130 000 mail requests. The relative effectiveness of different types of advertisement was evaluated through a series of tests. Table 6 summarizes the results of such tests, which measured the relative power of various advertisements aimed at creating demand for a free booklet. It can be seen that the newspaper advertisements produced very efficient results, with an advertising cost of only $0.07 for each response. The most successful in the series produced more than 1000 responses in the first ten days at an advertising cost of less than $0.03 per response. All respondents were sent literature, as well as a complete mobilization kit with motivational information, a *Preethi* sample and instructions for use. The total cost of distributing the kit, including postage, handling and advertising, was frequently less than $0.30.

Tests of direct-mail advertising also gave good results at low cost. Contraceptives and information were dispensed free and at low cost through the mail.

TABLE 6 Cost-effectiveness of advertising campaign for a free booklet by mail (Sri Lanka, 1974)

Medium	*Advertising costs (US dollars)*	*Number of responses*	*Cost per response (US dollars)*
Newspapers	1404	21 758	0.07
Radio	8110	25 047	0.32
Bus cards	166	401	0.41
All media	9680	47 206	0.21

Note: The $1404 used for newspaper advertising represents a fraction of total newspaper space used by the programme. Theme advertisements appeared frequently in a variety of newspapers. However, the figure of $8110 for radio represents the total allocation for that medium. A ban on contraceptive advertising by the Ministry of Broadcasting required the use of an extraordinary amount for a mail-order offer in order to gain exposure on the air. The ban was lifted in early 1976, paving the way for overt advertising of *Preethi* by radio.

It must be emphasized that the *Preethi* mail-order activities, and all other efforts undertaken throughout the launch period, represented harnessing of the indigenous resources. Structurally, none of the activities was new to Sri Lanka, although none had been used in the cause of family planning before.

SRI LANKA: CONCLUSIONS

The use of traditional, well established marketing systems for the advertisement and distribution of contraceptives provided a rapid, powerful impact. *Preethi* was accepted by 8% of the fertile couples in Sri Lanka during the first year of the programme at a cost of only $2.16 per acceptor. The programme brought about a fivefold increase in the use of condoms in less than three years. It should be noted that the marketing model produces lower unit costs with scale of use and over time. There is no doubt that oral contraceptives can also be handled by social marketing programmes and, although the Pill is a prescription item in Sri Lanka, a promising beginning has been made in marketing oral contraceptives.

BANGLADESH: EXPANDED APPLICATION OF SOCIAL MARKETING

The Sri Lanka programme was the first important test of social marketing of contraceptives through regular commercial channels, not calling into use business or government 'volunteers', or relying on agencies whose primary interests were other than commercial. It has become a model for other programmes, and the careful recording of the process leading to its success has become to some degree as important as the success itself.

In 1974, operating under the same programming and management philosophy and with the same basic goals, PSI, under contract to the government of Bangladesh and with USAID financing, initiated marketing research which led to another major social marketing programme: the highly successful distribution of *Raja* and *Maya* brands of condoms and oral contraceptives.

BARRIERS

The research design in Bangladesh was tailored to fit local conditions and was undertaken with the knowledge that:

* Bangladesh is one of the poorest and most crowded countries on earth, with a per capita annual income of $70 and with a population density of more than 1500 per square mile;
* overall literacy is about 20% and female literacy less than 10%;
* the Moslem religion is practised in a conservative way and women rarely leave their homes;
* the country presents unique physical barriers to distribution, with a deficient transportation and communications network and climatic factors resulting in a large percentage of the country being flooded for much of the year.

Therefore, Bangladesh was thought to provide a unique programming challenge, and there was speculation that if a social marketing undertaking could be made to work there, it could work anywhere. In the event, the research reported levels of awareness and approval of family planning consistent with levels in neighbouring countries. It confirmed a very low degree of practice but at the same time indicated what seemed to be a deep interest in and need for information about conventional contraceptives and other birth control methods.

Research also suggested that while retail and wholesale tradesmen were generally in favour of wider contraceptive distribution and promotion, some reluctance to display the products – especially condoms – could be expected.

PROMOTION

Consumer preference tests helped select the product names. The condom was finally called *Raja,* meaning king or ruler, a known and conceptually masculine word with the advantage that the package logo showing a stylized king as used on playing cards would be easily recognized even by those unable to read. *Maya,* selected for the oral contraceptive, is a pleasant and positive word, having among its meanings 'affection' and 'illusion'. As *Maya* is also used as a girl's name, packaging could feature a female face.

Because of several unique unknowns about the target population, the consumer market and the reach and influence of Bangladesh's mass media, a 'shotgun' approach to advertising and promotion was selected. All available methods were used during the introductory phase, with emphasis on radio and cinema (which do not rely heavily on audience education) and featuring, within both these media, carefully prepared original musical jingles. Press advertising, meant primarily to attract the favourable attention of opinion leaders and tradesmen, was initially designed to familiarize the reader with the package and brand names.

Point of purchase materials, posters, banners and booklets were distributed freely during the early launch period. Teams of promoters travelling the rural areas by bus, boat, cycle and rickshaw showed the labels, repeated the names and the basic message that *Raja* and *Maya* presented a safe, reliable, and low-cost choice to couples wishing to plan their families.

In the course of time, the advertising theme has switched away from packaging and brand name emphasis, and focused more narrowly on the combined theme of family happiness, financial security and good health. An attempt has been made to keep all advertising casual and pleasant in tone, stressing in positive terms the advantages of child spacing and small families as well as the features – quality, convenience and safety – of *Raja* condoms and *Maya* pills.

AVAILABILITY AND ACCEPTABILITY

National distribution began at the end of 1975. Priced to the consumer at a comfortable but significant US $0.01 per condom and US $0.05 per cycle of pills, the products rapidly achieved nationwide acceptance. Twelve months after their introduction, about one million condoms and more than 35 000 oral cycles were being sold per month. Using the Indian formula that 72 condoms provide one year's protection, it was estimated that about 200 000 couples were being served at that time.

By the end of 1977 distribution had more than doubled, to over 2 million condoms and 80 000-plus oral cycles monthly. One or both products were available in more than 32 000 retail outlets throughout the nation, and the names *Raja* and *Maya* were rapidly becoming generic terms for condoms and oral contraceptives. At this time, by official estimate, about one-third of the effective conventional contraceptive distribution in Bangladesh was being provided through the sale of *Raja* and *Maya*.

BANGLADESH: PERFORMANCE

The differences between evaluating a clinic-based family planning programme and a social marketing project have already been noted in relation to Sri Lanka. Social marketing programmes, by their nature, do not provide direct information about the total number of acceptors or continuation rates for the use of methods. They do offer, however, some unique advantages in evaluation:

* the fact that distribution is by sale, with payments received, provides a large measure of confidence in reported distribution statistics;
* there can be assumed to be a high degree of consistency between numbers of contraceptives purchased and numbers used;
* widespread and increasing acceptance of highly visible and often controversial advertising often indicates profoundly changing attitudes which, while not specifically measurable, may well be the beginning of a sharp increase in actual family planning practice.

Cost-effectiveness

In addition to sales statistics and distribution information such as number of outlets (which will eventually reach 50 000), costs are continually examined as a matter of course. During the year ending March 1977 the Bangladesh project spent a total of $650 000, including advertising, packaging, salaries, office expenses, overheads, etc. During the same period the income was about $90 000, leaving a deficit of $560 000. This amount can be taken as the actual programme cost. Enough contraceptives were sold during this time to provide full-time protection to 230 000 couples, hence the cost per couple-year of protection (CYP), excluding cost of donated contraceptives, was about $2.44. One year later, with 330 000 couples covered for a net cost of $465 000, this CYP figure had dropped to the remarkably low total of $1.41.

The Bangladesh social marketing programme is almost certainly providing the lowest per-couple service cost of any major contraceptive distribution effort in the world. Using the rough calculation that four years' protection is needed to avert one unwanted birth, current costs, including those of the donated contraceptives, work out to well less than $15 per birth prevented. And, as experienced in Bangladesh and Sri Lanka, these costs will become even lower as distribution expands and the cost of the marketing operation diminishes.

Towards self-sufficiency

Supporters of the social marketing concept point out that proven success and recognized potential for serving great numbers of both rural and urban people at low monetary and psychological cost present a powerful case for a much wider use of this method. They argue that consumers not only *prefer* to purchase contraceptives over receiving them free, but indeed in future will likely be *required*, through force of economic circumstances, to bear directly part, if not all, of the delivery cost of health, nutrition, family planning and other supplies and services to their community or home. Those opposed to social marketing often feel that there is something vaguely unsavoury about the commercial sector and immoral about selling essential goods – even at highly subsidized prices – to already needy people. Critics also point out that social marketing cannot directly serve the needs of the most needy, those with no disposable income. And locally there is almost always some degree of resistance, primarily among the educated urban wealthy, to mass media presentation or discussion of such 'intimate' subject matter as family planning or contraception.

CONCLUSIONS

As the argument continues, more enlightened governments, such as that in Bangladesh, recognizing that all segments of the population must be served *now*, are actively encouraging programmes of social marketing to supplement the more traditional clinical and other public sector programmes. Projects have been or are being carried out in Kenya, Colombia, Jamaica, El Salvador, Nepal, Korea, Haiti, the Philippines and others, in addition to Sri Lanka and Bangladesh.

Success in these projects varies, but one fact is emerging clearly: contraceptive distribution programmes based on use of commercial techniques and using the consumer goods delivery system available in every country, given the flexibility to operate dynamically in the marketplace, can effectively and inexpensively supplement national family planning programmes.

Social marketing is here to stay. What remains is to implement social marketing programmes in more and more countries, to perfect and refine the approach as it is adapted to each area. And the need of the hour, as in all family planning endeavour, is to do so without reservation and with all possible speed.

Bibliography

Black, T. R. L. and Harvey, P. D. (1972). The commercial distribution of contraceptives. In M. Potts and C. Wood (eds.). *New Concepts in Contraception.* (Lancaster: MTP Press)

Black, T. R. L. and Harvey, P. D. (1976). A report on a contraceptive social marketing experiment in rural Kenya. *Studies in Family Planning,* **7** (4), 101

Franda, M. F. (1972). Marketing conditions in India; the Nirodh program. *American Universities Fieldstaff Reports,* **16** (8), 1

Gupta, D. R. (1972). The battle of the population bulge. *Victor-Bostrum Reports,* **16,** 7

Jones, G. W. and Selvaratnam (1972). *Population Growth and Economic Development in Ceylon.* (Colombo: Hansa Publishers Ltd.)

Korten, D. C. (1975). Population program 1985: a growing management challenge. *Studies in Family Planning,* **6** (7), 178

Kotler, P. and Zaltman, G. (1971). Social marketing: an approach to planned social change. *Journal of Marketing,* **35,** 3

Nortman, D. (1975). Population and family planning programs: a factbook. *Reports on Population/Family Planning.* No. 2, 7th Edition

Piet, D. L. and Hendrata, Lukas (1974). Karet KB and Jamu: an integrated approach to condom marketing. *International Development Review,* **4,** 2

People (1975), **2** (4), Issue devoted to reviews of contraceptive distribution

9

Self-sufficiency in family planning – Japan*

Chojiro Kunii

MY INVOLVEMENT IN FAMILY PLANNING BEGINS 154
OBJECTIVES OF THE FAMILY PLANNING MOVEMENT 154
ESTABLISHMENT OF THE JAPAN FAMILY PLANNING ASSOCIATION (JFPA) 155
Forming the Study Committee on Family Planning 156
The effects of the newsletter 157
DISTRIBUTION OF CONTRACEPTIVES 158
DEMAND FOR CONTRACEPTIVES EXPANDED 159
COMMUNITY-BASED DISTRIBUTION (CBD) SYSTEM 159
Development of education materials 160
Interpersonal network 161
Establishment of related organizations 161
CURRENT STATUS OF THE JFPA 162
CONCLUSIONS 162
STATISTICAL INFORMATION 163

*First published in 'Proceedings of the Third Consultative Meeting for Integration', April 1978

MY INVOLVEMENT IN FAMILY PLANNING BEGINS

One day in the autumn of 1953, I was asked by an officer of the Ministry of Health and Welfare (MHW) to implement the dissemination of family planning ideas and various contraceptive methods throughout Japan on a voluntary basis. At that time the Japanese government was alarmed by the rapid increase in the number of induced abortions. In 1952 the government had decided to initiate a national family planning campaign for preventing abortions and distributing contraceptives among couples, for the reasons that induced abortion incurs harm to the mother's health and also was generally considered immoral.

Based on this decision, a nationwide family planning campaign was begun at 700 governmental health centres. However, the results were very discouraging; it was found to be a rare thing for people to visit health centres to consult on family planning methods or to get contraceptives.

Because of such poor results, the government thought that it might not be suitable for government institutions to be involved in such a delicate and private matter and began to seek another way to conduct a family planning movement. Finally the government decided to establish a private organization to do this work. This was the background of the government's proposal to me.

OBJECTIVES OF THE FAMILY PLANNING MOVEMENT

Having heard the government's proposal, I thought it over carefully and discussed family planning with my colleagues and, finally, I decided to accept the proposal. But, as I knew relatively little about this social and individual problem, I began to study contraception, abortion and other population problems. I visited various agencies, such as the Institute of Population Problems, Institute of Public Health, Population Problems Research Council of the Mainichi Newspapers and other related agencies to collect the relevant books, data, and information. I also visited several pioneers in the field of population and family planning and listened to their opinions. These people included Mrs Shidzue Kato, Dr Kan Majima, Dr Yoshio Koya, Dr Tenrei Ota and Dr Juitsu Kitaoka, all of whom played an active role in this field especially after World War II.

However, one crucial and basic problem remained after this elaborate preparation. I could not understand why family planning had to be promoted among the people. One of the experts explained that family planning was the only solution to the overpopulation problem which became serious after World War II and that overpopulation was the main reason for Japan's poverty at that time.

Another expert said that family planning was needed mainly for the prevention of induced abortions, that is, for the protection of the mother's health. It was the growing tendency after the enactment of the Eugenic Protection Law in 1948, which legalized induced abortion not only for medical reasons but also socioeconomic reasons, that the number of induced abortions had increased greatly year by year. Induced abortion was, in those days, not only very dangerous to the mother's health, but it also caused serious side-effects and in the worst case the mother's death. In order to alleviate this situation it was necessary to diffuse family planning concepts and methods among couples throughout the country.

Which position should I take and emphasize? This was the first and most important question for me. Japan was defeated in World War II and had more than 80 million people living in four narrow islands (total area of 360 thousand square kilometres). Such problems as food shortage, unemployment, stagnation of economic production and disease were seriously undermining the Japanese people.

Under such circumstances I could easily understand the significance and implications of 'population control' which economic leaders, national planners and businessmen were insisting upon. However, I was very sceptical about people's reactions to family planning for these reasons. It seemed very difficult for individual people to connect the macro-level problems of food shortage, unemployment and economic stagnation with the practice of family planning.

Sex is a basic element in human existence. It is entirely an individual and private matter, and as family planning is directly connected with this, it stands aloof from persuasion with such macro-level reasons. If we consider our own life more precisely, we come to conclude that people rarely decide to have or not to have children by considering economic development and the future of the nation. I discussed the above notion frankly with the people at MHW and they fully agreed with my opinion. As a result the single and clear objective of 'protection of the mother's health' was established, though the Council on Population Problems (under direct jurisdiction of the government) insisted upon a different view that 'protection of the mother's health' was not strong enough to persuade people and it was better to include another objective, i.e. 'population control for national development'.

ESTABLISHMENT OF THE JAPAN FAMILY PLANNING ASSOCIATION (JFPA)

On request from the MHW it was necessary to form a strategy for family planning activities. I then submitted a proposal which included a plan to establish a Japan Family Planning Association (JFPA). The establishment of this association also had a strategic purpose. The proposal included a statement on the objectives of family planning activities along with my own thoughts and explained the role of the new organization as follows:

* the association would publish a monthly organ and distribute it to all the health centres (700), the persons in charge of the health departments at the prefecture, city, town and village level (3500), midwives, public health nurses and the persons in charge of health care in various private organizations (planned total circulation was 20 000). In this weekly newsletter, information concerning family planning would be delivered in plain language;
* the association would distribute contraceptives (such as condoms, jelly, etc.; at that time oral pills did not exist as a contraceptive) of good quality and at a cheap price;
* the association would conduct training (including in-service training), seminars and conferences for family planning workers at the local and central levels;
* the association would produce and distribute educational materials relating to family planning.

My proposal was accepted by the government (MHW) without any modification. The government agreed to conduct family planning activities according to the outline of this proposal through a private organization.

But great difficulties awaited me. I found that MHW had no budget for my activities. So I had to seek money for the programme's operation on my own. I was able to solicit only 200 000 yen. That was far short of the amount needed to publish even the first issue of the family planning newsletter. However, I began to issue 3000 newsletters every month. Original programmes had to be cut down owing to shortage of funds. The association had no full-time staff at that time. I worked intensively, even on Sundays and holidays.

At that time I was a Director of the Japan Association of Parasite Control and lived on that salary. People at the MHW felt sorry for me because I had to work with no funds, and often asked various companies (such as pharmaceutical, life insurance and milk-producing companies) to run advertisements in our newsletter. This kind of informal request is very effective in Japan. I refused to run advertisements of contraceptives at that time as I was afraid of misunderstandings among people that the JFPA was only a retailer for contraceptive manufacturing companies.

Forming the Study Committee on Family Planning

Thus, I began my voluntary activities by editing and publishing a monthly newsletter entitled 'Kazoku Keikaku (Family Planning)' on a small scale in

April 1954. In order to collect data and information as well as basic ideas on family planning for the newsletter, I organized the 'Study Committee on Family Planning', the members of which were demographers, doctors who were interested in family planning, heads of health centres, junior officers of the MHW and journalists. These members were all young and fresh and the meetings which were held once a month, with enthusiastic discussions, often continued until midnight.

Occasionally public health nurses, midwives or opinion leaders who were actively engaged at the grass-roots level participated in the discussions. One public health nurse said, 'We are taught that, as public health nurses, our purpose is to work for improvement of people's health. This is the main reason that I became a public health nurse. And I thought that I would be very happy if I could help people from this point. If the aim of family planning is social and economic development we don't want to promote family planning.' Another public health officer from a village said, 'I think it is not true that overpopulation is the sole cause of unemployment, hunger or economic stagnation. Such reasons seem to be an excuse for poor governmental policy.'

This Study Committee made a great contribution to the development of our movement, refining the philosophy, developing educational materials, and producing various strategies. I myself was much impressed and gained a detailed knowledge of family planning from the discussions. In this way the inexperienced JFPA could devise strategies and gain new information.

The effects of the newsletter

I had to make strenuous efforts to publish the 'Kazoku Keikaku (Family Planning)' newsletter. To collect accurate information the MHW helped me considerably. Such information lent authority and credibility to the newsletter. All the members of the Study Committee on Family Planning became regular contributors. Before printing, any inconsistent points among writers were thoroughly discussed. I also planned slogans to express family planning objectives. Some examples are as follows.

'To protect mothers' health'

'To bear and raise a healthy child'

'To make a happy family'

A round table discussion, short stories, poems and comics were added, but without detracting from the dignity of the newsletter. The publication of this newsletter contributed greatly to the promotion of our activities:

* Through editing the newsletter we came to understand the current conditions of family planning and maternal and child health (MCH) activities that had been carried out at the local level.

* We were directly informed about existing problems with MCH activities or demands from mothers at the local level. Based on this information I could plan on what to do next.
* The newsletter also played an important role in communicating relevant information all over the country.

DISTRIBUTION OF CONTRACEPTIVES

During the 6 months that passed from the first publication of the newsletter, many kinds of letters and requests from readers were delivered to my small office. The demand for cheap contraceptives of good quality was found to be an urgent one for many readers. At that time poor quality contraceptives such as condoms with defects were sold at pharmacies. I planned to distribute condoms to health centres, family planning workers, local municipalities and factories at a low price.

In the autumn of 1954 I visited the Okamoto Gomu Company, which was the biggest condom maker in Japan, accompanied by Senator (Mrs) Shidzue Kato. The objective of this visit was to negotiate the sales of condoms to us at a special wholesale price. It was part of a strategy to have Senator Kato, who was not only a famous member of the House of Councillors but a great pioneer in family planning, accompany me. The negotiations succeeded. The company promised to sell us condoms at one-quarter of the market price. That gave me great pleasure. If the idea met with success as originally intended, the JFPA could earn a considerable amount of money even if condoms were sold at half price. With this money I wanted to employ more people, increase the circulation of the newsletter, train FP workers and produce educational materials such as films, filmstrips and leaflets.

However, we needed to do more work before selling condoms. First of all, a new package had to be designed for our condoms. This needed to be somewhat 'elegant' because of the rather poor image associated with condoms. (They had been used as a protection against venereal disease.) The second idea was the insertion of a leaflet into the package on the objective of family planning (mother and child health care), in poetic form for easy understanding. A third idea was that we call the condoms that were to be sold by the JFPA 'FP' condoms. In order not to be copied by other dealers, we succeeded in registering it as a trademark.

We realized these preparations for sales in a very short time and from the next month we began to advertise the condoms in our newsletter. Before long, one women's club in Nagano Prefecture made an advance order of a large quantity of condoms. A certain publishing company of a women's magazine also ordered many of them. The welfare section of a mining company ordered condoms for thousands of couples working for the company.

DEMAND FOR CONTRACEPTIVES EXPANDED

In 1956 the MHW started a programme called the 'Special Project for Diffusion of Family Planning'. This programme focused on poor couples. The government (MHW) had appropriated about 60 million yen to this project. Local governments added an equal amount for the project. In all, a total amount of 120 million yen was provided for this new programme (including the expense for contraceptives).

At that time a person at the MHW said to me, 'We are very sorry that we could not help your activities at the beginning. Now your efforts will be repaid'. By this time the MHW had approved the JFPA and permitted us to sell condoms and other contraceptives. In addition, the MHW indirectly suggested to local governments (prefecture, city, town and village) to purchase contraceptives (mainly condoms) as well as educational materials from the JFPA and to distribute them to the eligible couples through home visits. These home visits were conducted by family planning workers (private midwives) who lived in each local community. A small amount of money was given to midwives for their work.

Before actual distribution all eligible couples in a target area were given group guidance by public health nurses who worked for local municipalities or health centres. Through this counselling, couples learned about family planning ideas and methods from films, filmstrips, pamphlets and other means. After this kind of group guidance, individual guidance by the midwives followed. Condom use was gaining and demand was increasing year by year.

COMMUNITY-BASED DISTRIBUTION (CBD) SYSTEM

With Japan's economic development during the late Sixties, the income of poor families had also increased. As a result, the central government decided to curtail the special project for poor couples. However, the demand for contraceptives at the grass-roots level was still very high.

Thus, after the withdrawal of central government funding, local health centres or municipalities bought contraceptives directly from the JFPA and distributed them to the people. In this case couples used to buy the contraceptives with their own money. Some of the practising midwives living in local areas voluntarily served as distributors. These midwives could make a profit of 30–35% on the contraceptives sold. Besides the profits from sales, they were also provided with a small amount of money through the governmental MCH programme for their home visits (US $2.50 per visit, as of 1978).

As circumstances changed in this way, the JFPA also organized a mobile unit in 1966 and tried to meet local demands. This mobile unit, stocked with many contraceptives and educational materials, made rounds to local municipalities, health centres, midwives, public health nurses, etc. With this system the JFPA was able to supply contraceptives and educational materials as well as hold film shows and group counselling in joint cooperation with the local governments or health centres.

The community-based distribution system has strengthened the economic stability of the JFPA. With this system the JFPA could not only expand its community activities but gain more profits from selling contraceptives and educational materials.

Development of educational materials

We made great efforts to develop educational materials for FP workers at the community level. A serious problem for FP workers was the lack of educational materials of good quality. Firstly, we asked Dr Yoshio Koya to write a short essay to explain family planning in plain language. We produced a small pamphlet which gained a very good reputation among the people. We also produced wall charts, films, and filmstrips in rapid succession.

One interesting incident occurred in 1955 regarding our first film, 'Basic Knowledge of Birth Control'. The two major themes of this film were: (1) to illustrate the reproductive systems of the male and female using various charts that included human anatomy, and (2) to teach the mechanism of pregnancy and methods for its control. After its completion I visited the Tokyo Metropolitan Police Board (MPB), which was a big purchaser of our condoms, to show the film (the MPB had many young eligible couples). I planned to sell some copies of the film to the police. However, after the preview, I was called by the chief of the discipline section who looked at me sternly. He said to me, 'We never buy that kind of film because the film shows the pubic hair of the female. It violates discipline regulations'. The MHW became upset over this charge and got into a dispute with the MPB over the matter.

In the end, the MHW and the JFPA were defeated in the dispute. We deleted the controversial segment and put a revised version on sale the second time. However, fortunately the dispute about hair between government officers created such a sensation that as a result our film sold very well. A total of 200 copies were sold. Consequently, the JFPA earned a large amount of money.

Interpersonal network

In expanding some kind of activity, a group of experts whose thinking is consistent is needed as a core. This kind of core group is indispensable in creating an international network. For this purpose we have held various kinds of meetings and conferences. They are as follows.

National Conference on Family Planning and MCH – once a year (since 1956)
About 2000 people participate at this conference in which special lectures and presentations concerning the experiences of activities are given and discussed. On this occasion a Health and Welfare Minister's Award is given to FP workers or doctors who have made distinguished contributions to family planning programmes. All expenses for the conferences are borne by private organizations, which are also responsible for programme planning.

Local Study Meeting – once a year (since 1957)
There are two types of local study meetings. One is the joint meeting of several prefectures (en bloc) with similar geographical characteristics. Another is the individual meeting held in a single prefecture. In both cases expenses for the meeting are borne by private organizations and the programme is prepared jointly by the local government and our organization.

Seminars (since 1956)
There are several kinds of seminars such as the training seminar for the qualification of FP workers (twice a year; about 100 participants each), refresher courses for FP workers, seminar on marriage counselling (for doctors and nurses), etc.

All preparation and management of these seminars and meetings are conducted by the JFPA under the joint auspices of both the central and local governments. Through these seminars a nationwide interpersonal network for family planning has developed in Japan. And this network has produced good results.

Establishment of related organizations

The JFPA cooperated in the establishment of several related organizations both financially and through the supply of human resources. The ideas, costs and staff needed for the establishment of the National Federation of Maternal and Child Health Centres were borne by our association (1962). The Japanese

Organization for International Cooperation in Family Planning (JOICFP) was also established and assisted by our association (1968). At present these organizations work in cooperation with each other (they are located in the same building).

CURRENT STATUS OF THE JFPA

In Japan, 70% of couples (both rural and urban) have only two children. Thus we can say that contraception is considered among all couples as one of the necessities of life. The infant mortality rate is nine per thousand, ranking as one of the lowest in the world. The average lifespan for male and female is 72 and 78 respectively. This ranks among the top rates in the world. In the light of these conditions, the central focus of family planning activities cannot but change from that of 20 years ago.

(1) Since 1977 the Japanese government has commissioned the JFPA to conduct genetic counselling in connection with family planning activities. To implement this, the government has provided the JFPA with a subsidy totalling 16 million yen annually. This has been the first grant from the government to the JFPA since its establishment. As the amount is not enough to cover all the expenses for the genetic programme, the JFPA will make up the deficit. Genetic counselling is conducted every day (part of the expenses is charged to the individual). We plan to make a nationwide network for this activity.

(2) In 1974 the IUD was legalized by the government and the association is now planning to open a clinic for IUD and FP counselling in Tokyo. Now the JFPA has branches in Akita, Hyogo, Ehime, Fukuoka, Miyazaki, and Okinawa prefectures. By assisting these branches' activities the association tries to disseminate family planning ideas in each area.

CONCLUSIONS

I believe that the following components are very important in expanding a family planning programme. First in importance is the mutual cooperation of the government, scientific experts and private organizations. In other words, the private organization must play an active part in the cooperation between the government and scholars and serve as a link between the two. Secondly, a self-reliance system facilitates innovative and flexible growth which a voluntary organization needs. Based on its economic self-reliance system, the JFPA is working its way to a new future with the assistance of the Japanese government and the scholars concerned.

STATISTICAL INFORMATION

TABLE 1 Ideal number of children by age of wife (percentage) (1973)

Wives' ages (years)	*Don't want children*	*One child*	*Two children*	*Three children*	*Four children*	*More than five*
20–24	1.1	4.2	47.6	40.7	3.7	2.1
25–29	0.7	4.2	37.6	48.8	5.7	2.6
30–34	0.4	2.7	37.9	45.4	8.8	2.4
35–39	0.5	1.4	35.2	45.8	11.3	1.9
40–44	0.8	2.3	28.5	47.4	11.6	3.1
45–49	0.9	1.5	20.1	44.9	17.1	7.5

Source: Family Planning Public Opinion Surveys; Population Problems Research Council; the Mainichi Newspapers

TABLE 2 Numbers of reported induced abortions (1949–76)

1949	246 104	1962	985 351
1950	489 111	1963	955 092
1951	638 350	1964	878 748
1952	805 524	1965	843 248
1953	1 068 066	1966	808 378
1954	1 143 059	1967	747 490
1955	1 170 143	1968	757 389
1956	1 159 288	1969	744 451
1957	1 122 316	1970	732 033
1958	1 128 231	1971	739 674
1959	1 098 853	1972	732 653
1960	1 063 256	1973	700 532
1961	1 035 329	1974	679 837
		1975	671 597
		1976	664 106

Source: Statistics and Information Division; Health and Welfare Minister's Secretariat

TABLE 3 Percentage of contraceptive users and non-contraceptive users (1950–75)

Year	*Currently practising*	*Previously practised*	*Have no experience*	*Other, No answer*
1950	19.5	9.6	63.6	7.3
1952	26.3	13.8	54.9	5.0
1955	33.6	18.8	41.6	6.0
1957	39.2	17.3	38.3	5.2
1959	42.5	20.2	33.0	4.3
1961	42.3	26.1	28.5	3.1
1963	44.0	19.0	29.8	7.2
1965	55.5	16.5	26.8	1.2
1967	53.0	19.2	23.1	4.7
1969	52.1	19.1	19.3	9.6
1971	52.6	20.2	16.8	10.4
1973	59.3	22.0	15.1	3.6
1975	60.5	21.0	13.3	5.2

Source: Family Planning Public Opinion Surveys; Population Problems Research Council; the Mainichi Newspapers

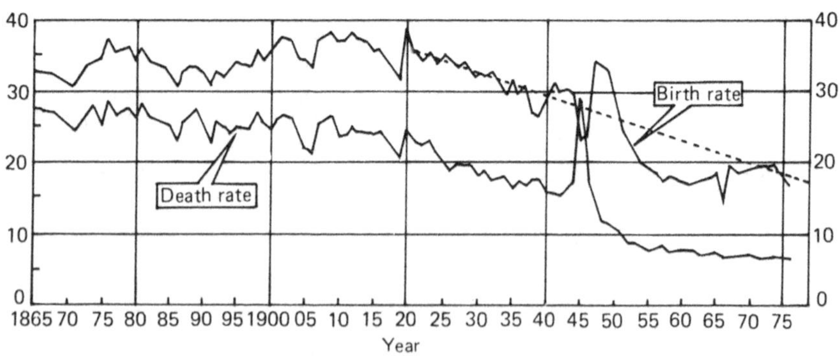

Figure 1 Birth and death rates in Japan

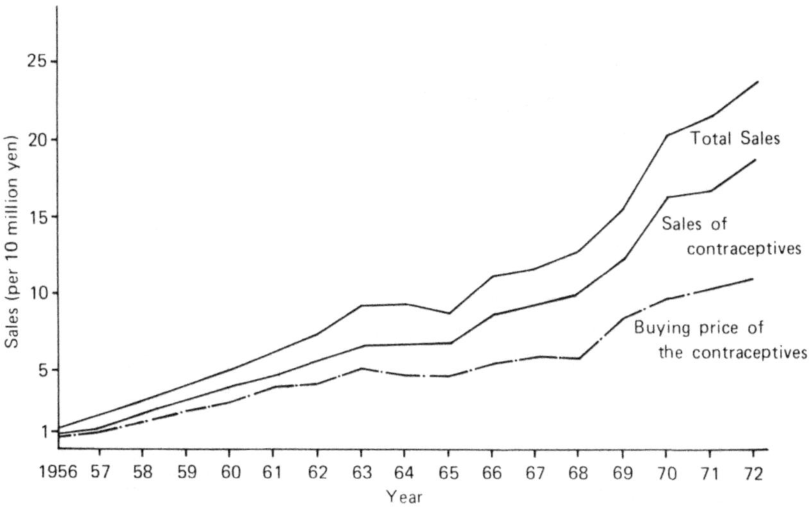

Figure 2 Sales by Japan Family Planning Association (1956–72)

TABLE 4 Attitude towards family planning (percentage)

Year	*Good thing*	*Indifferent*	*Not a good thing*	*Never thought of it, don't know*	*Others, No answer*	*Total*
1950	60.7	—	15.0	18.6	5.7	100.0
1952	65.0	—	11.6	20.6	2.8	100.0
1955	67.4	—	10.8	18.9	2.9	100.0
1957	72.0	—	9.2	6.8	12.0	100.0
1959	74.2	—	8.8	5.9	11.2	100.0
1961	69.1	—	7.6	8.0	15.3	100.0
1963	88.0	1.9	0.6	6.1	3.4	100.0
1965	87.5	1.7	0.8	6.3	3.4	100.0
1967	84.9	2.8	1.3	7.5	3.5	100.0
1969	84.6	2.3	1.5	7.8	3.7	100.0
1971	85.4	3.0	1.1	7.4	3.1	100.0
1973	87.0	2.5	1.0	7.1	2.4	100.0
1975	86.5	3.0	0.7	7.4	2.4	100.0

Source: Family Planning Public Opinion Surveys; Population Problems Research Council; the Mainichi Newspapers

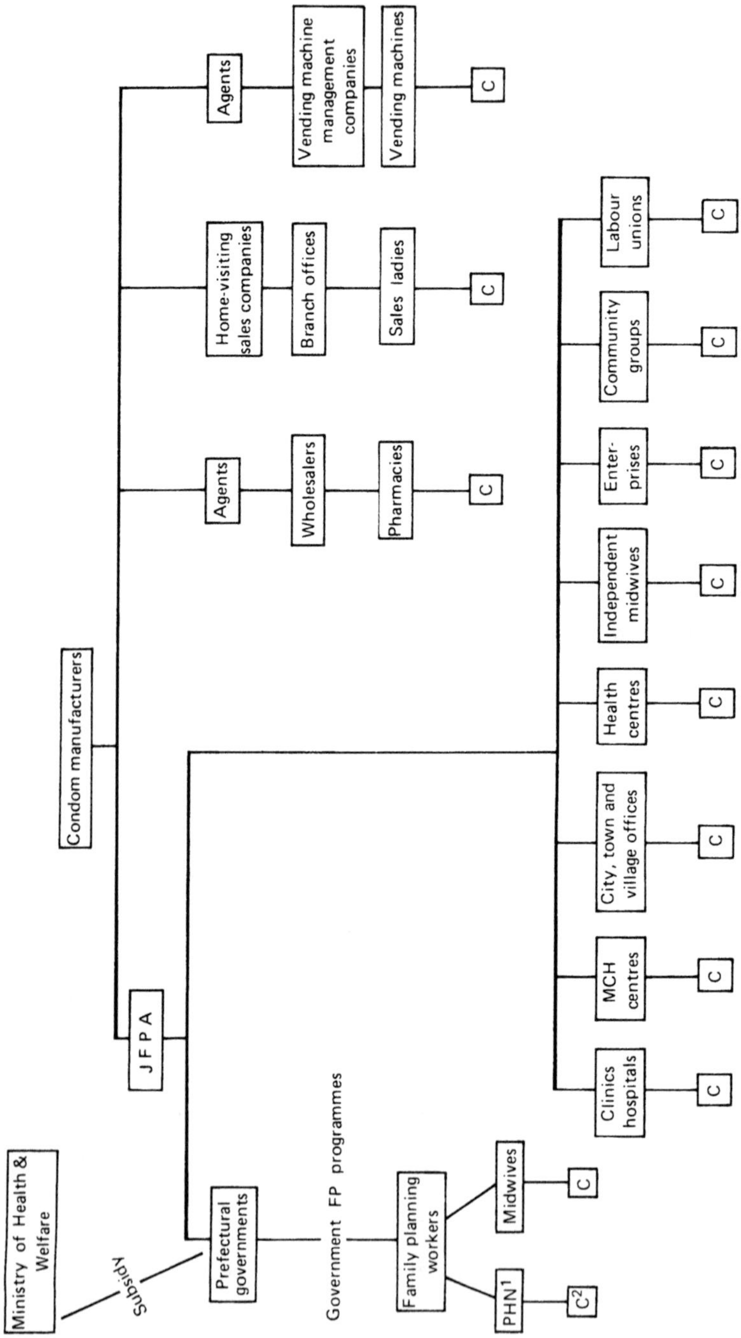

1. PHN = Public Health Nurse
2. C = Consumers

Figure 3 Distribution channels of condoms in Japan

TABLE 5 Budget for family planning by the Ministry of Health and Welfare (1952–76)

Year	*Total amount (one million yen)*	*Equivalent in $US (thousand dollars)*
1952	21.2	58.9
1953	39.3	109.2
1954	28.9	80.3
1955	58.7	163.1
1956	58.5	162.5
1957	71.8	199.4
1958	72.5	201.4
1959	54.1	150.3
1960	47.7	132.5
1961	53.8	149.4
1962	55.9	155.3
1963	62.7	174.2
1964	66.4	184.4
1965	34.3	95.3
1966	60.8	168.9
1967	66.9	185.8
1968	70.8	196.7
1969	81.4	226.1
1970	81.2	225.6
1971	88.8	246.7
1972	97.2	270.0
1973	110.0	366.7
1974	128.7	429.0
1975	155.2	517.3
1976	140.7	469.0

(1) Figures indicate the total amount of budget allocated to the Ministry of Health and Welfare for family planning. Local prefectures usually add the same or double the amount distributed to them from the Ministry of Health and Welfare depending on the item, and therefore, the actual total expenditures for the country as a whole are about 2.5 times as much as the indicated figures.

(2) On 14 February 1973, the foreign exchange rate changed in Japan. Until 1972 one dollar was equal to 360 yen, while after 1972 one dollar is equal to 300 yen.

TABLE 6 Annual budget of Japan Family Planning Association

Fiscal year (April–March)	*Amount (Unit: 10 thousand yen)*
1954	(estimated) 100
1955	(estimated) 500
1956	1144
1957	2140
1958	3209
1959	4228
1960	5221
1961	6475
1962	7294
1963	8446
1964	10 200
1965	9600
1966	10 800
1967	11 800
1968	13 000
1969	15 500
1970	19 000
1971	23 500
1972	24 500
1973	28 000
1974	36 500
1975	43 000
1976	47 500
1977	53 000

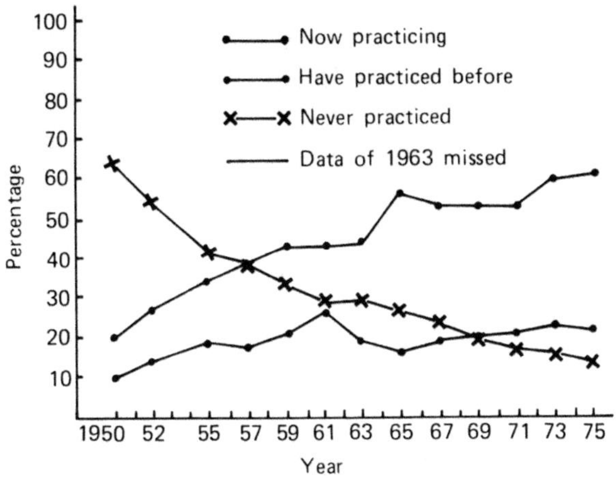

Figure 4 Result of family planning public opinion surveys

Bibliography

Japanese Organization for International Cooperation in Family Planning (1977). *Fertility and Family Planning in Japan.* Japanese Shipbuilding Industry Foundation

Japanese Organization for International Cooperation in Family Planning (1977). In: C. Kunii and T. Katagiri (eds.). *Basic Readings on Population and Family Planning in Japan.* (Tokyo: J. OICFP)

Koya, K. (1963). *Pioneering in Family Planning.* (New York: Population Council)

Muramatsu, M. (1967). *Japan's Experience in Family Planning – Past and Present.* (Tokyo: Family Planning Federation of Japan)

SECTION THREE

Barriers and Bottlenecks

Future developments in contraceptive research can be predicted within broad limits. A number of modest but useful developments may still take place in relation to existing methods, but fundamentally new techniques are likely to take many years to develop and introduce.

One element in fertility control which seems likely to remain unchanged in the foreseeable future is the resort to induced abortion which, whether legal or illegal, is common and appears to follow a predictable pattern in relation to fertility control.

Menstrual regulation is a simple, safe technique that could meet many of the demands for early abortion, but which for political reasons unrelated to the technique itself, remains controversial in a number of countries.

The need for female sterilization outstrips the capacity to provide them. It is the family planning method that demands most skill and equipment for its performance. Therefore, research to improve and simplify the operation is of particular significance.

Basic research is the only way of improving family planning techniques in the long term. Unfortunately, in recent years the investment in research relevant to contraceptive development has declined in actual terms. This is a situation which needs to be remedied.

Although the international investment in family planning has now risen to several hundred million dollars a year, the total investment of the United States of America – the most generous country in this field – is still, over a ten year period, less than 2 weeks' expenditure on health care by the US.

10

Female sterilization

Pouru Bhiwandiwala

INTRODUCTION	174
WHO WANTS STERILIZATION?	175
The right to choose	175
WHY IS STERILIZATION NECESSARY?	176
Benefits	177
Demographic impact	177
HOW CAN STERILIZATION BE TAKEN TO THE PEOPLE?	178
Reaching the people	178
WHAT ARE THE BOTTLENECKS?	179
Bureaucratic barriers	179
Organizational problems	180
WHAT IS AVAILABLE TODAY?	181
Sterilization programme status	182
WHAT LIES AHEAD?	183
New developments	183
Reversal of sterilization	184
TO STERILIZE OR NOT TO STERILIZE?	184

INTRODUCTION

Voluntary sterilization has gained recognition in many parts of the world, and is now regarded as an intrinsic and necessary component of any family planning programme. In recent years, the increased utilization of this method to control fertility has been most dramatic – from 2 million couples in 1950, to 20 million couples in 1970, and 80 million couples in 1978. The family planning tide is flowing strongly towards sterilization (Potts, 1976), and the world-wide surge of support is continuously growing. Voluntary sterilization has been eagerly accepted in whichever country it has been made available, irrespective of geographical, cultural and economic differences. The increased demand can be partly attributed to the marked change in the prevailing attitudes of the political and religious leadership and the medical profession. However, every effort must now be directed to overcome bureaucratic barriers and make sterilization services available to those who need it the most.

Currently, a large variety of female sterilization techniques are being used, which suggests that none of them is perfect. The recently developed methods are relatively simple, safe, and effective, but the search goes on for a non-surgical procedure which is not totally doctor-dependent. This is absolutely vital, as most developing countries are overburdened with health problems, and cannot afford to spare a large slice of medical skills for sterilization services. One of the arguments which is foolishly but consistently offered to justify the non-availability of sterilization is the high cost relative to other contraceptive methods. This fallacy must be rectified, and the cost-effectiveness of the method by way of averted births and total years of protection needs to be emphasized. Controversies about the acceptability of the procedure have been ended once and for all by the intense demand of couples who have gone to great lengths to avail themselves of this service. In some poor regions of the world, a woman faces more than a 10% chance of dying from a high parity pregnancy and childbirth. The villagers may be illiterate, but they are intelligent enough to choose to live and care for their existing children, if given the opportunity.

Recently, a lot of publicity has been focused on human rights. Surely an individual has the right to have as many children as she wants – and yet the simple option of sterilization is denied to so many. Instead of concentrating on taking services to the people, there is a tendency in some countries to develop a maze of rules and regulations to 'protect' the woman. Although abuse of sterilization does exist to some extent, the bureaucratic barriers do very little to prevent it, and it is not clear whether they are supposed to safeguard the user or the provider. There has been a rapid transition from the time when sterilization was only available for *medical indications,* to the present situation where it can be obtained *on request* in many countries. It is estimated that by 1985, 200 million couples will elect to use sterilization, and at least half of them will be in the developing countries. The current demand considerably exceeds the availability of services, and this gap is likely to widen at an accelerated pace unless rapid and effective measures are taken to increase the resources and overcome the bottlenecks.

WHO WANTS STERILIZATION?

Millions of couples around the world have demonstrated that voluntary sterilization is a most acceptable solution to the problem of fertility control. The benefits of this method are so substantial that individuals and families have put themselves to great inconvenience in an effort to obtain these services. In some places where sterilization was not easily available, women have travelled to another country to undergo this procedure. The response in the rural areas has surpassed even the most optimistic expectations. Women along with their entire families have walked long distances to the camps, where sterilizations are provided on a temporary basis by a visiting mobile team. On some occasions, the demand has been so overwhelming that women have had to wait for 2 or more days – but very few have turned back without the procedure. This offers the most convincing proof of the acceptability of sterilization at all socio-economic and cultural levels.

The change in attitudes of policy-makers, administrators and the medical profession has significantly contributed to the increased availability and consequent acceptance. Another major factor is the development of simpler and safer techniques which are performed under local anaesthetic on an outpatient basis, thereby eliminating the social and economic problems associated with hospitalization. Expanding health services have improved the survival rates of children, and sterilization is an acceptable option after the desired family size is achieved.

The right to choose

The World Population Plan of Action (1974) states that 'all couples and individuals have the basic right to decide freely and responsibly the number and spacing of their children'. The principle should not exist only on paper, but every individual must be allowed to exercise this right. It can only be accomplished by providing 'on request' services, instead of setting up elaborate eligibility criteria. Most couples make their own decisions concerning all-important personal matters such as marriage, career, investments, etc. and nobody interferes or raises an eyebrow. Since couples understand their own circumstances, needs and desires better than anyone else, is it not logical to assume that they should be allowed to choose when to be sterilized?

TABLE 1 Estimated number of couples using voluntary sterilization by country in 1977

Country	*Number of sterilizations (in millions)*
China	35
India	22
Asia (excluding China and India)	3.5
United States	9.5
Europe	5.5
Latin America	3
Canada	1
Africa	0.5
Estimated world total	80

WHY IS STERILIZATION NECESSARY?

A family planning programme without the option of sterilization is like a car with a rundown battery. It is for a good reason that the IPPF panel of experts has recommended that 'both male and female sterilization should always be made available as part of a comprehensive family planning service'. It not only fills a vacuum but also adds a much-needed impetus to the programme. Reversible methods of contraception are absolutely desirable and essential, but have their limitations. Generally, women complete their desired family size when they are in the late twenties or early thirties, and that leaves them with an additional 10 to 20 years of fertile life. The use of reversible contraceptives during this period is not only inconvenient, but there is a high possibility of an unplanned pregnancy. In addition, the side-effects associated with prolonged use of some contraceptives must be taken into account. There is an increased risk of cardiovascular disease in women over 35 years of age who are on the Pills, especially if they smoke cigarettes. Reversible methods are essential for postponing and planning pregnancies, whereas sterilization is far more suitable for family limitation – therefore both methods are necessary and complementary to each other.

Benefits

Voluntary sterilization is a vital preventive health measure, and the benefits are actually measurable. A significant reduction in maternal morbidity and mortality has been demonstrated by preventing the high order pregnancies and births which are associated with increased risks as described in Chapter 2. Illegal abortions have claimed innumerable lives and often caused permanent damage to those who have survived this ordeal. In addition, the treatment of these unfortunate women places a tremendous strain on an already overburdened health system. A substantial number of these abortions are likely to be high order pregnancies which could be avoided by the proper use of voluntary sterilization, thus saving numerous human lives as well as medical resources and manpower.

The risks of the procedure are minimal, whereas the advantages are immense. Sterilization is a one-time method, which does not require sustained motivation, periodic check-ups, or dependency on contraceptive supplies. It is extremely cost-effective considering the number of years of protection that it provides. The risks have been further minimized by the use of local anaesthetic and improved techniques. Complications, if any, are rarely life-threatening, and the incidence ranges from 1–2%. The long-term effects of psychological disturbances and menorrhagia (excessive blood loss through the vagina) are rather doubtful, and a definite association with sterilization has yet to be confirmed. Considering the benefit–risk ratio, the advantages of sterilization far outweigh the adverse effects, and contribute significantly to the improvement and promotion of family health.

Demographic impact

Although it is impossible to pinpoint the impact of any one factor on the fertility rate, there is enough evidence to indicate that the increased acceptability and availability of voluntary sterilization in recent years has played a major role in slowing the world population growth. The demographic impact of sterilization depends essentially on the age and parity of the women accepting this method. However, it has a high use-effectiveness and each procedure is expected to avert 1.5 to 2.5 births. Dr R. T. Ravenholt has estimated that by making sterilization fully available to populations in developing countries, the fertility of women over the age of 30 could be reduced by about 25%.

HOW CAN STERILIZATION BE TAKEN TO THE PEOPLE?

The urgent necessity today is to make sterilization available to all people throughout the world, and extend the services to the rural areas where they are needed the most. This would involve an immense effort on the part of governments, donor agencies, voluntary organizations and the medical profession. The attitude of the government varies in different countries ranging from active provision of services, to indifference and even open hostility. Encouragement, financial support and technical assistance from donor agencies have served to promote sterilization in countries which do not have the resources, trained personnel and facilities. For fiscal year 1978, the US Agency for International Development has allocated $25 million for voluntary sterilization, and other funding organizations have also committed substantial amounts. However, it is the local voluntary groups led by a few courageous individuals who are ultimately responsible for the rapid spread and availability of sterilization in many countries. In recent years, the medical profession has yielded to public pressure, and an ever-increasing number of physicians are performing the procedure.

Reaching the people

Millions of the world's poor want to control their fertility, but it is the availability of sterilization that will ultimately determine its use. Information and promotion among users (potential and current) and the medical profession are essential components of a sterilization programme as discussed in Chapter 7. Urban areas do not pose a major problem, as it is relatively simple for physicians, clinics and hospitals to add sterilization services to the existing facilities. The real challenge lies in reaching the rural areas, and a number of successful approaches have been implemented. Of these, the sterilization camps have proved to be the most acceptable and cost-effective. There is a considerable variation in the implementation as indeed there should be, and experience alone will tell what is suitable for a particular region. The sterilization camp is planned well in advance and, via various communication channels and personnel, the message is extensively spread among the neighbouring and remote communities. The response in most areas has to be seen to be believed. The women arrive at the campsite either alone, in groups, or accompanied by the entire family. Modes of transport include bullock-carts, animal-drawn carriages, cycle-rickshaws, public transportation wherever available, but by and large the villagers depend on their own two feet. Very often, the campsite resembles the scene of a festivity or the platform of a busy railway station. The operating room is set up in the village meeting-hall, classroom, local clinic, tent or whatever is available. The sterilizations are performed by a visiting medical team, and the physicians generally use a technique with which they are familiar and comfortable.

It is hoped that more countries will develop this camp approach, but obviously it may not be suitable for every region. Other efforts to reach the rural areas include the provision of sterilization services at rural health centres and clinics. This is accomplished either by training the local doctor if available, or arranging for physicians from neighbouring cities to periodically visit and perform procedures at the centre. Almost all community-based systems providing reversible contraceptives, include referrals for sterilization. Private family planning hospitals set up by non-profit organizations in several countries are providing inexpensive, high-quality services for surgical methods of fertility regulation. It may be a worthwhile experiment to extend loans to cover start-up costs for similar services in rural areas. The availability of male sterilization at railway stations, in mobile vans, discarded buses and bamboo booths temporarily set up in any crowded area, certainly did wonders for popularizing the procedure. Hopefully, in the near future, the female sterilization technique will be further simplified, thereby offering far more options for taking services to the people.

WHAT ARE THE BOTTLENECKS?

Bureaucratic barriers

Although religious and cultural restrictions do lower the acceptance of sterilization, motivated individuals often have a way of getting around them.

However the legal, administrative and organizational barriers are the major obstacles to providing and accepting sterilization services. The present situation is a tremendous improvement over the past, and there is every reason to be optimistic about the future. Only six countries in the whole world now legally prohibit voluntary sterilization – Burma, Greece, Portugal, Italy, Somalia and Spain. Several countries either have ambiguous laws, or specific legislation just does not exist. According to legal authorities 'what is not prohibited is permitted' and therefore sterilization is performed openly. As the governments become involved in the provision of sterilization services, there is a directly proportional increase in official red tape. The requirement of informed consent by the spouse is mandatory in many countries. Various eligibility criteria for women requesting sterilization are still in existence. Until recently, 'the rule of 120' was observed in the United States, Europe and Australia – the woman could obtain sterilization only if her age multiplied by parity amounted to 120 or more. In some places, authorization by a medical committee or special board is required. Rules have recently been enforced in the United States requiring a waiting period of 30 days following the woman's request for sterilization. In addition, informed consent cannot be obtained while the woman is in labour, or if she is undergoing an induced abortion.

Organizational problems

In most countries, the facilities for sterilization are inadequate but the demand continues tô grow. In places where women are required to be hospitalized following sterilization, only a fraction of those requesting the procedure actually obtain it, due to the excessive demand on beds. The obstetric services are so busy managing deliveries, that they tend to neglect the long-term needs for birth control. Prolonged waiting times of up to 6–12 weeks to obtain a sterilization in a hospital or clinic, and long queues at sterilization camps are fairly common in many countries. The shortage of resources is further compounded by the lack of trained physicians to perform the procedure. In Bangladesh, non-doctors (trained village women) successfully perform sterilization under supervision, and in Iran, qualified midwives are providing this service. At the current level of technology it appears that dependence on the physician will continue until simpler methods are developed. However, some of the tasks presently performed by doctors (prescription of Pills, insertion of IUDs, etc.) could be safely delegated to non-doctors, enabling more efficient utilization of physician time.

Obviously the cost of sterilization is higher than any other contraceptive method (even though it may be the cheapest in the long run), and this does pose a problem when financial resources are limited. In developing countries, the average cost of a minilaparotomy ranges from $14 to $20, and a laparoscopic sterilization would vary from $25 to $35. Laparoscopic equipment not only involves a large initial investment (about $3000), but requires provision for maintenance and repair, and special training for the entire medical team. However, in some circumstances, this can prove to be more economical in the long term. In the United States, one day of hospitalization could cost over $150 (exclusive of all other expenses for surgeon's fees, operating room, etc.), and a capital investment in equipment would be cost-beneficial if the need for hospitalization were eliminated. On the other hand, in a developing country, an entire rural health centre could be constructed for the price of the laparoscopic equipment. Therefore, the decision concerning capital investment has to be made on an individual basis to fit the situation.

WHAT IS AVAILABLE TODAY?

Sterilization has evolved from a hysterectomy (removal of the uterus) to a ten-minute outpatient procedure. The introduction of the Pomeroy method of tubal occlusion (which leaves the uterus intact), is a major landmark. Initially the procedure was offered only for medical indications, but a few courageous farsighted physicians also performed it on women who were over 35 years of age and had six or more children. It is only recently that the arbitrary rules of age and parity have been relaxed and the individual's choice is being respected. However in some parts of the world, women are still undergoing hysterectomy as a contraceptive measure in spite of the higher health risks, when sterilization is not available due to religious or legal barriers.

The principle of female sterilization very simply is to prevent the sperm from meeting the egg which is released every month. Since fertilization takes place in the fallopian tubes of the woman, an occlusion of the tubes either by cutting them or blocking the lumen will keep the sperms apart from the egg. Human imagination has run wild in discovering different ways of cutting and blocking the tubes. The Pomeroy technique which involves tying and cutting off a portion of the tubes has stood the test of time, and is probably the most widely used procedure. According to some enthusiastic supporters of this method, all it requires is 'a knife, a piece of string, and the physician's fingers'. This is obviously an oversimplification, but it is basically true. The tubes can also be occluded by burning them with an electric current (electrocoagulation), applying a silastic band (Falope ring), or a tubal clip. Currently the best results are being obtained with the Falope ring, and this method of occlusion is rapidly gaining popularity.

In order to gain access to the fallopian tubes, five different approaches can be used – laparotomy, minilaparotomy, laparoscopy, colpotomy and culdoscopy. *Laparotomy* is the traditional method which requires an incision similar to other abdominal surgery. This approach is gradually becoming obsolete for interval sterilization, but it remains the method of choice in women who have recently delivered as the tubes are easily accessible at this time. *Laparoscopy* involves the use of an optical instrument introduced into the abdominal cavity. In a *colpotomy,* the tubes are approached through a small incision in the vagina, and in *culdoscopy* an optical instrument is introduced through the vaginal cul-de-sac. *Minilaparotomy* requires a very small suprapubic incision, and is easy to perform with ordinary surgical instruments. This is by far the most popular and practical method available today.

Sterilization programme status

The highest number of voluntary sterilizations in the world have been performed in China, India and the United States. Asia accounts for the bulk of the sterilizations, while Africa lags far behind (Table 1). The Chinese family planning programme relies heavily on surgical sterilization and clearly leads the world in this method. In one commune, 48% of the protected couples had used female sterilization. High social and peer pressure, together with increased availability of female sterilization has led to an enormously successful programme. In India, during fiscal year 1976–77, over 2 million female sterilizations were performed as a result of pressure exercised by the government. In Bangladesh, since 1975, a surge of sterilization programmes and campaigns have greatly increased the number of female acceptors. By 1985, the government plans to have 500 health facilities equipped with sterilization services, which are becoming increasingly popular in this Muslim country. In Singapore and the Philippines, of the total number of sterilizations performed in 1976, 96% and 81% respectively, were on females.

The Middle Eastern and North African countries have varying policies regarding female sterilization – in Tunisia, the national family planning programme is supporting these services; in Egypt, only private institutions offer sterilizations; and in Turkey, female sterilization can only be performed for medical indications. The incidence of female sterilization in sub-Saharan Africa is the lowest in the world. In the Latin American countries, the legal status of voluntary sterilization remains questionable and varies greatly. Puerto Rico has the most successful voluntary female sterilization programme and in both Central America and Colombia, this method is widely available. In Brazil and Chile, female sterilization can only be obtained through private physicians, and in Argentina it is illegal. In Eastern Europe and the USSR, sterilization is almost impossible to obtain. Some countries like France, Belgium, Poland and Switzerland have no laws regarding sterilization, whereas Czechoslovakia and Norway require a review board to authorize a sterilization procedure. The German Democratic Republic allows female sterilization but forbids male sterilization. In Italy, Greece, Spain and Portugal, sterilization is illegal. In England, voluntary sterilization is widely available. In the United States, sterilization is becoming exceedingly popular among married couples, more than 29% of whom are covered by either male or female sterilization, and it is expected that female sterilization will overtake oral contraceptives as the method of choice.

WHAT LIES AHEAD?

New developments

Although major advances in technology and equipment have been achieved, a single 'ideal' method is still not available. Resources for research in sterilization are limited, but a number of promising techniques are currently being developed. Considerable attention is now being focused on non-surgical and temporary (or reversible) sterilization methods. The use of quinacrine for chemical sterilization has the outstanding advantage that it is very simple to perform and is similar to inserting an IUD. Quinacrine pellets are introduced into the uterine cavity through an inserter, and no special instruments are required. It acts by causing scarring of the tube at the uterotubal junction, but requires three insertions at intervals of 1 month in order to be effective. If this technique proves to be successful, it could be administered by trained paramedical personnel. Methyl-2-cyanoacrylate (MCA) is also a blocking agent which is delivered transcervically and has a similar mode of action. Silicone rubber plugs which are introduced into the tubes via the uterine cavity have the advantage of being a surgical as well as reversible sterilization method. The use of cryosurgery to produce endometrial ablation is currently being studied. Systematic non-surgical methods being tested include immunization against specific hormones or unique tissue antigens. Reversible techniques of female sterilization which show some promise include silastic caps which cover the fimbrial ends of the tubes; ovariotexy (the ovary is covered with a silastic sheet); burying the tube; and silicone rubber plugs. Endoscopic equipment is being constantly improved and costs are being lowered, but this will not serve the extensive needs of the developing countries.

Reversal of sterilization

This issue has recently gained considerable attention. Some misguided enthusiasts strongly advocate that the possibility of reversal should be widely publicized in order to increase the acceptance of sterilization. *This would certainly be a sad mistake and should be discouraged.* Every woman accepting sterilization must be made to understand that it is a permanent method. If however, due to some misfortune or special circumstances she needs to have her fertility restored, she should then be given the option for reversal. The success rate (determined by a uterine pregnancy) using the conventional technique of tubal anastomosis is not very encouraging. A survey in the United States showed that it was successful in less than 30% of carefully selected women. The probability of success is considerably increased by the use of microsurgery, but this requires expensive equipment and extensive training. The frequently quoted statistics, giving a success rate of 90%, have only been obtained by a few specialists, who have practised the technique for several years (initially on laboratory animals) using sophisticated operating microscopes worth thousands of dollars. This result cannot necessarily be replicated by a gynaecologist who occasionally performs the procedure. It would be ideal if the government of each country would set up a 'Sterilization Reversal Centre' with essential equipment and one or two trained specialists. Some reversible techniques of sterilization are currently being developed, and it is hoped that they will become a reality and will set the stage for a sterilization revolution.

TO STERILIZE OR NOT TO STERILIZE?

The time has now come to shed all arbitrary eligibility criteria, and provide sterilization on request. The main obligation of the physician should be to ensure that the woman is making a free choice without pressure and is not mentally disturbed, and also to determine that both partners understand that the method is irreversible. The maze of bureaucratic rules and regulations should be gradually dissolved, and all efforts must be concentrated on making sterilization available to the millions who want it. According to the famous biochemist Albert Szent Gyorgi, 'Today's question is not whether there is life after death, but whether there is life after birth'. Sterilization is an important option which can help to make every child a wanted child. It is now the leading method of fertility control, and the acceptance is expected to increase steeply in the next few years. Barriers and bottlenecks are being overcome, and there is every reason to be optimistic for the future.

Bibliography

Green, C. P. (1978). M/F sterilization. *Population Reports*. Special topic monographs, 2

McCann, M. F. and Bhiwandiwala, P. Is minilaparotomy appropriate in the United States? *Advances in Planned Parenthood*. (In press)

Potts, M. (1976). Bureaucratic barriers to sterilization. *Draper World Population Fund Report*, 3

Ravenholt, R. T. (1976). World epidemiology and potential fertility impact of voluntary sterilization services. In: Marilyn E. Schima and Ira Lubell (eds.). *New Advances in Sterilization*. (New York: The Association for Voluntary Sterilization, Inc.)

Speidel, J. J. (1976). The future of female sterilization technology. *International Journal of Gynaecology and Obstetrics*, **14**, 17

11

Menstrual regulation

Elton Kessel

INTRODUCTION	187
Differences from abortion	188
Similarities to abortion	189
Nomenclature	189
PERFORMANCE	190
Research	190
Safety	191
Efficacy	194
ACCEPTANCE	195
COST-EFFECTIVENESS	198
SUMMARY	199

INTRODUCTION

Menstrual regulation (MR) is a medical or surgical procedure performed on woman with delayed menstrual periods who do not wish to be pregnant. The most common procedure is vacuum aspiration of the uterine cavity using a small plastic cannula. It is frequently performed within 2 weeks of expected onset of menses, when the diagnosis of pregnancy cannot be reliably determined.

The idea of aspirating a uterus with a small diameter cannula is not new. It was described in 1872 by Queen Victoria's obstetrician who referred to the procedure as 'dry cupping'. It followed on from the quasi-medical use of leeches applied to the skin in the hope of producing menstruation from the uterus. In 1924 a well-known gynaecologist told the Philadelphia Obstetrical Society that he routinely performed the operation on an out-patient basis without anaesthesia and, in subsequent years, it received occasional attention in the medical literature.*

Modern menstrual regulation dates from 1970 when Karman developed the transparent, flexible, polyethylene cannula with a rounded tip and two triangular apertures and adapted the 50 cc plastic hand syringe for use as a vacuum source. The timing was opportune. There was growing concern over a world-wide epidemic of abortion and the development of menstrual regulation services promised to reduce the demand for legal abortion and, under some circumstances, illegal abortion as well.

Differences from abortion

The distinction between menstrual regulation and abortion can be made on several counts, the most notable being the uncertainty of an existing pregnancy. Although pregnancy tests, such as radioimmunoassay, which are accurate within 14 days of an expected period, do exist, they are unlikely to be readily available to most of the world's populations within the next decade. In the absence of facilities for microscopic examination of the uterine aspirate, the proportion of menstrual regulation procedures that terminate pregnancies can only be estimated on the basis of number of days' delay in menses and the outcome of the pregnancy test. This proportion may also be affected by a woman's age, parity, lactation and recent use of steroidal contraception. The legal implications of the uncertainty of an existing pregnancy are of particular interest, because opinion has held that laws relating to abortion are not applicable to menstrual regulation.

There are also important physiological differences between MR and abortion at 7 to 12 menstrual weeks gestation. The cervix is generally not dilated for MR, but must be dilated for the later gestations. The products of conception increase in mass geometrically with gestation and, in contrast to

* For an excellent history see *Population Reports*, Series F Nos. 2 and 3, 1973

later abortion, an incomplete menstrual regulation procedure is unlikely to be life threatening. These differences have implications for the level of professional training required for menstrual regulation and for abortion.

Similarities to abortion

The demographic transition from high to low fertility in a population probably can not be accomplished without heavy reliance on abortion, and the effectiveness of induced abortion – whether legal or illegal – in controlling rapid population growth has been demonstrated on numerous occasions. According to certain analysts, population growth must be decelerated in order to permit the economic well-being of a society. Their view would appear to be substantiated by the drop in birth rates (the effect of abortion) in Japan and certain Eastern European countries and the subsequent rise in their standard of living as well as by the place which illegal abortion seems to have played in the economic and demographic changes in nineteenth century America.

When post-conceptive procedures are initiated, the sudden drop in rates of maternal morbidity and mortality and the concomitant decrease in infant and child mortality rates and illegitimate births are impressive. By contrast, contraceptive methods are more slowly adopted and in few or no countries has fertility decline been solely due to improvements in contraception.

Nomenclature

It seemed that each new practitioner of the procedure had his own name for it – menstrual regulation, menstrual extraction, endometrial aspiration, mini-suction, mini-abortion, the Karman technique – to name just a few. But it was difficult to know what to call a procedure when its purpose was not known – removal of a conceptus, or removal of the endometrium. It is necessary to have a name broad enough to include both surgical and medical procedures, particularly as since 1972 there have been hopes that a self-administered abortifacient could be developed. The term *very early abortion* is unsuitable as some operators would have to report a proportion of 'very early abortions' performed on non-pregnant women! The term *menstrual extraction* seems best reserved for vacuum aspiration procedures performed before a delay in menstruation. This procedure has been advocated by some womens' groups in the USA as a matter of convenience to shorten menstrual periods. While the term *menstrual regulation* is less precise, it focuses on the objective of the procedure, which is to give the woman a regular menstrual period. The term also had the advantage of avoiding the negative connotations of the word abortion.

PERFORMANCE

The assessment of menstrual regulation involves a number of different factors. The frequency with which it may be necessary to perform the procedure, its relationship to contraceptive use, and the possibility of pregnancy continuing if the uterus is evacuated early in gestation, need to be studied. It is also necessary to evaluate different types of equipment, the training that is required, and to determine if paramedical personnel can perform this procedure safely.

Research

Menstrual regulation was chosen as one of six major study areas by the International Fertility Research Program (IFRP) in 1971, primarily because of the promise of a self-administered prostaglandin as an abortifacient with an acceptable level of side-effects. The studies of vacuum aspiration for menstrual regulation are now essentially complete, although we still await a practical non-surgical technique of treating menstrual delay.

The first systematic studies were begun by the International Fertility Research Program (IFRP) in 1972. The research to be undertaken was crucial in the light of:

* an increased number of contraceptive users in many countries with consequently more contraceptive failures and more women requesting treatment of their missed period;
* a general increase in acceptance of abortion and the hypothesis that early termination of a suspected pregnancy, before the diagnosis can be reliably made, may involve less risk of physical and psychological trauma to the patient than waiting until a definite diagnosis is possible;
* the suggestion that a very small cannula with vacuum aspiration is safe and effective treatment;
* the development of abortifacients, such as the prostaglandins, that might be practicable for self administration to induce uterine bleeding shortly after a missed period.

Some difficulties were anticipated before the initiation of IFRP studies. For example, numerous gynaecologists had had unreported experiences of attempting to remove an ovum in early pregnancy with a small curette without dilation of the cervix, only to have the pregnancy continue. But, apparently, few of these physicians had attempted to use the more recently introduced plastic cannula and vacuum aspiration technique for this purpose. The Joint Program for the Study of Abortion (JPSA) reported that complications increased with gestation, except before the seventh week from the last menstrual period, when complications were higher than in that week. It was suggested that this might be due to dilation of the still unsoftened cervix. But there was also the possibility that with the newer vacuum aspiration technique dilation of the cervix would not be necessary and that a smooth decline in complications with shorter gestations would be found. While it was recognized that some unnecessary procedures would be performed on non-pregnant women, it was thought that, depending on its magnitude, this risk would be acceptable, relative to the higher risk of complications with induced abortion at later gestations. Determining this relative risk was one of the primary objectives of the research protocol. The IFRP Menstrual Regulation Study Protocol collected information on the characteristics of women having the procedure, on the type of procedures and on complications at the time of the procedure, and at a two-week follow-up visit. The diagnosis of pregnancy was documented by the presence of villi on microscopic examination of aspirated uterine contents.

It became apparent early in the study that the intrauterine administration of prostaglandins, while effective, could not compete with the low level of side-effects of vacuum aspiration. As a result, the preponderance of studies have been of the vacuum aspiration technique.

A standardized form was used to collect the data. Early studies in countries where abortion was illegal were limited to cases with a negative pregnancy test. Later, large-scale studies were initiated in a few centres to include cases beyond two weeks delayed menses in order to try to document whether complications fell smoothly with shorter intervals of gestation. Comparative studies with random allocation of techniques to subjects were initiated for different vacuum sources, vacuum pressures and cannulae sizes, utilizing the same basic data collection instrument as in straight studies. Table 1 shows the number and distribution of menstrual regulation studies and procedures with the vacuum aspiration techniques.

Safety

Menstrual regulation by vacuum aspiration is safe. About eight complaints or complications occur per 100 procedures and only approximately half of these are significant complications. The incidence of complications increases steadily with the number of days of menstrual delay. The complications of

TABLE 1 Distribution of menstrual regulation studies

Country	*Number of centres*	*Initiation date*	*Number of cases*
Americas			
Chile	1	July 1974	391
Ecuador	1		
USA	9	October 1972	4506
Europe			
England	3	October 1972	1035
Hungary	1	February 1974	94
Yugoslavia	2	November 1974	398
Middle East			
Egypt	2	June 1973	967
Iran	7	June 1973	2971
Africa			
Ghana	1	January 1975	250
Nigeria	1	January 1975	455
Asia			
Australia	1	May 1977	
Bangladesh	2	July 1974	1394
India	15	November 1972	5543
Indonesia	6	February 1974	1250
Korea	1	February 1973	55
Malaysia	1	June 1974	288
Pakistan	1	February 1974	14
Philippines	4	June 1973	487
Singapore	1	March 1973	4230
Sri Lanka	1	August 1975	140
Taiwan	1	January 1977	500
Total	**62**		**24 968**

Source: International Fertility Research Program, July 1977

MR are lower than for routine abortion at 7 to 8 weeks gestation. For women with a positive pregnancy test there is no question that the procedure should be performed at the first visit as a very high proportion of such women are pregnant. For those with a negative pregnancy test, the saving in major complications by delaying the procedure for one week is modest (Figure 1). Significant complications per 100 women would be reduced from 3.9 to 3.7.

The operator must be able to interpret the risk of complications to the patient. Her decision to have the procedure at the first visit or later will no doubt be influenced by her level of anxiety about a possible pregnancy and the inconvenience and expense of a second visit. This will vary greatly for different cultural settings.

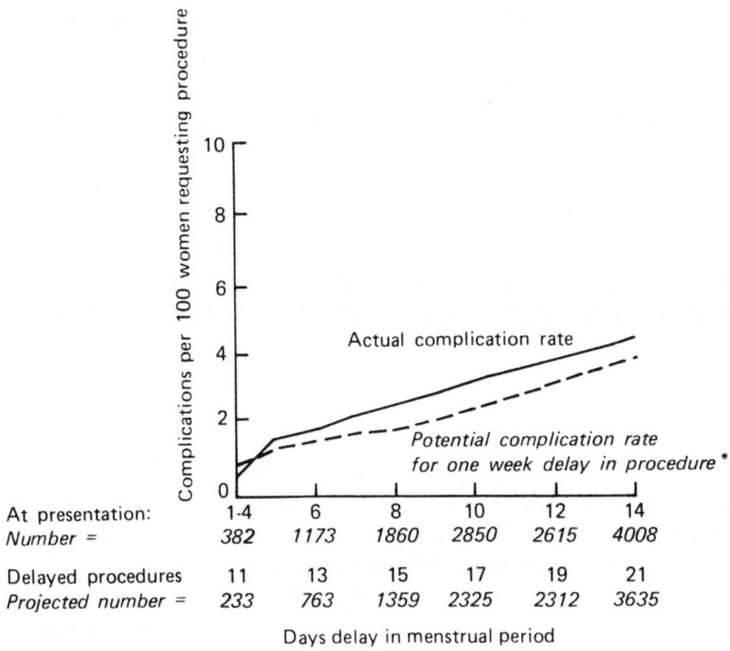

Figure 1 Complication rates

*The potential complication rate in women with negative tests which are delayed one week uses the same denominator (number of women requesting treatment) as for the actual complication rate, although the actual number of procedures performed is reduced by the number of women who experienced a menstrual period

There are wide variations in reports of complications, including retained products requiring repeat vacuum aspiration. Carefully controlled studies have not been conducted for menstrual regulation to determine the role of variation in skill of the operator in various rates of complications. Such studies have been conducted for first trimester abortion and they do show considerable variation in complications among operators, such variation being greater than that attributed to the use of rigid or soft plastic cannulae. It is likely, therefore, that much of the variation in complication rates reported for menstrual regulation is also related to operator skill and experience.

Because menstrual regulation is still a relatively new method of treatment for large segments of the world's population, there has been no systematic evaluation of the possible serious, delayed complications that might result with repeated use. It has been postulated that induced abortion can affect the outcome of future pregnancies as a result of Rhesus immunization and of prematurity which may be one consequence of cervical injury sustained at the time of dilatation and curettage. These complications should not occur with menstrual regulation because Rh immunization* is unlikely to be associated with the procedure and dilation of the cervix is minimal, if at all needed.

There are additional benefits of some importance that accrue to women undergoing menstrual regulation. Microscopic examination of the endometrium may allow for specific diagnosis and treatment. If products of conception are not identified in the tissue evacuated from the uterus and the pregnancy test remains positive, an ectopic pregnancy may be diagnosed early.

Efficacy

The efficacy of menstrual regulation as a method of contraception must be measured in terms of (a) the individual procedure needed by a couple using some form of contraceptive and of (b) menstrual regulation used as the sole means of fertility regulation. Menstrual regulation is highly effective as evidenced by the fact that there were only 113 patients who still had a positive pregnancy test at a 2 week follow-up visit out of 13 178 procedures reported to the IFRP (with a menstrual delay of 14 days or less). This gives a failure rate of about 1%, compared with a reported 0.5% for first trimester abortion.

A wide variation of failure rates for menstrual regulation have been reported in the medical literature. These may be related to the experience and skill of the operator in performing the procedure and the adequacy of the vacuum produced by the equipment which is used. In a study of menstrual regulation procedures performed by registered nurse-midwives, a failure rate of 2.1% was reported for the first 142 cases. After additional training was provided by an experienced gynaecologist, the failure rate dropped to zero for the next

* Rh immunization of a pregnant woman with a Rh negative blood type can occur if she carries a fetus with a Rh positive blood type. The antibodies formed by the mother can destroy the fetal blood cells and result in fetal complications or stillbirth. The earliest gestation at which the Rh factor has been demonstrated in fetal blood is at $7\frac{1}{2}$ menstrual weeks. Rh immunization has not been reported under seven menstrual weeks gestation.

571 cases. Faulty surgical technique and inadequate care of equipment were responsible for the initial failures.

For the woman using MR as her only means of fertility regulation repeat procedures will be needed. Empirical data indicate that women 30 years of age or under will require approximately three procedures per year to remove a pregnancy, and women over 30 two. To compare the efficacy of MR with other methods of contraception one may multiply the failure rate (1%) by the number of required procedures per year, giving rates between 2 and 3 per 100 women per year, similar to failure rates for IUDs and other effective methods.

When MR is used as a backup for contraceptive methods, the combination results in essentially no failures. The exact failure rate of the two (presumably independent) methods would be the product of the two failure rates. When MR is combined with a straightforward mechanical method of contraception, such as the use of condoms, the combination is one of outstanding safety and freedom from side-effects for the user.

To measure the efficiency of menstrual regulation, one must examine its rate of failure and the proportion of procedures performed on non-pregnant women. Since the failure rate is negligible, the major determinant of efficiency becomes the treatment that was, after all, unnecessary. The physiological, pharmacological and pathological status, as well as the length of amenorrhoea, affect the proportion of women with less than 14 days delay in onset of menses who are indeed pregnant. Assuming an average cycle of 28 days, then among women with 7 days of menstrual delay, 52.6% are pregnant and by 14 days of menstrual delay, the rate is 84.1% in IFRP studies.

In summary, while women should be informed of possible complications, they can be assured of the relative safety and effectiveness of this early post-conceptive method of fertility regulation.

ACCEPTANCE

Menstrual regulation is gaining acceptance in an increasing number of medical centres and among practitioners in many countries. When women learn of the existence of a responsible service providing abortion or menstrual regulation, they invariably tend to avail themselves of it in preference to other more dangerous options.

Early reports from India indicate slower acceptance in a rural community clinic than in urban community clinics in West Bengal. In Bombay, a community clinic situated within walking distance of the population it serves shows greater utilization of menstrual regulation services and at fewer days of delay than a large teaching hospital clinic. In the Model Clinic in Dacca, MR is the most common *first* method of fertility control accepted. Menstrual regulation services with varying criteria of delayed menses are openly offered in many other countries, even those with restrictive abortion laws. These include clinics in Indonesia, Malaysia, Thailand, the Philippines, Taiwan, Mexico, Ghana and Nigeria. There is a tendency in some clinics, especially those in countries where abortion is legally restricted, to extend the acceptable period of delayed menses to three or more weeks, while still referring to the procedure as menstrual regulation.

Systematic studies of menstrual regulation as a new fertility regulation service are difficult in those countries where the legal status of the procedure is still uncertain. However, individual documented cases provide an impressive record. For example, a single practitioner in South East Asia who learned to do the operation in 1973–74, began by performing approximately eight MR procedures a month, but at the end of 1977 was doing six to eight a day. In 2000 consecutive procedures the general practitioner had had one perforation of the uterus which required hospital admission and laparotomy. The normal practice followed is to sedate the woman with Valium 5 mg about 15–30 minutes prior to the procedure which is performed in a small, clean room. A sterilizer for boiling the speculum is the only additional requirement. The operation normally takes 3–5 minutes and after waiting in the corridor for about 15–30 minutes the woman finds her own way home. She is given an antibiotic cover. The country concerned is one where routine abortion is only available on strictly health indications, but menstrual regulation is becoming increasingly acceptable.

In one Roman Catholic country of 40 000 000 population it is estimated that approximately 10 000 menstrual regulations are performed each year. Responsible doctors, eager to see some solution to the appalling public health problems presented by illegal abortion, are offering MR increasingly freely. In some places, experienced and practised physicians have been teaching others to perform the operations. The experience has been that this type of training is welcome. A large number of practitioners performing perhaps 10 or 20 procedures a week, can make a significant contribution to a community of several million people. It is hoped that within the foreseeable future, where such services exist, there will be a demonstrable decline in the toll of women entering public hospitals with the consequences of illegal abortions.

In one of the richer, but still developing countries of Asia, a single menstrual regulation clinic was set up in 1973. Today, it is performing approximately 200 procedures a month and has been able to repay the small venture capital necessary to create the clinic. What is particularly impressive is that this example of success has been copied by other practitioners in the capital city and it is now known that there are at least 10 such clinics, each with a similar turnover of cases. In another Asian country a single practitioner does 20–30 MRs a day. Women travel many hours by public transport to seek the services and some arrive a full six hours before the clinic opens its doors. Patients stand in a queue waiting for the operation and the line extends up to the two tables where the operations are performed.

In the examples given, the responsible doctors see menstrual regulation not as an isolated entity, but as part of family planning and whenever possible have offered post-abortal contraceptive advice. For many women the procedure has also been an introduction to family planning practice. Conversely, for those who have been using a method of contraception and have been faced with an unlucky pregnancy, it has added to the creditability and the acceptance of the method.

The International Pregnancy Advisory Service (IPAS) has taken a lead role in developing and distributing MR kits (Table 2) and in training, organizing and setting up not-for-profit clinics. In India, Taiwan and Hong Kong the kits are manufactured indigenously. There is apparently less of a demand for the modified 50 ml syringes in industrialized countries, possibly because vacuum aspiration equipment is freely available.

TABLE 2 Menstrual regulation distribution – International Pregnancy Advisory Services

		MR kits distributed [1]			
Region	*Number of countries*	1975	1976	1977	1978 [1]
Americas	12	585	197	1850	2765
Europe	11	493	689	846	377
Middle East	8	5332	437	161	1
Africa	10	296	6986	941	2818
Asia	18	15 928	1910	11 121	5375
TOTAL	59	22 634	10 219	13 919	11 336

[1] Data refers to imported kits and not to local manufacture
Source: International Pregnancy Advisory Services, 123 West Franklin Street, Chapel Hill, North Carolina 27514, USA (unpublished data)

Conferences have had a major effect in disseminating information and supplies that lead to menstrual regulation services. The Menstrual Regulation Conference in Honolulu in December 1973 did a great deal to disseminate the technology. After the Menstrual Regulation conference in Dacca in February 1975, menstrual regulation studies and distribution of menstrual regulation kits increased in Bangladesh. A Pathfinder meeting at Airlie House, Virginia helped disseminate the technique in Latin America. The variety of cultural settings in which these kits have been distributed and menstrual regulation services provided, suggests the very wide acceptability of the procedure.

COST-EFFECTIVENESS

The cost-effectiveness of menstrual regulation in a family planning programme must be evaluated in terms of the specific goals of the programme. The financial cost is low, when compared with induced abortion. MR is safely performed on an outpatient basis in a treatment room and requires only 5–10 minutes of professional time. Preliminary experience with nurses trained to perform the procedure has been encouraging; their rates of failures and complications are no higher than those for physicians.

One of the outstanding advantages of menstrual regulation is that the procedure is of sufficient simplicity that it can be made available, even in the poorest of communities, on a financially self-sufficient basis. For example, in one South East Asian agricultural community the procedure is currently offered at US $6. In the Indian subcontinent traditional indigenous practitioners who have learnt the procedure are offering it at US $1–3. In another country, in poor urban areas and in the villages, one system of pricing is US $3 for every week of delay after the menstrual period. The practitioners who charge fees of this type still make a significant additional income and, in some cases, may well be in the process of doubling their income.

In a public family planning programme where part of the budget is allocated to attracting clients, a proportion of the menstrual regulation service costs might be considered a recruitment cost. In several international studies it was found that more than 90% of the menstrual regulation patients subsequently accepted IUDs or oral contraceptives. In one of the services mentioned earlier all the women having MR receive an IUD at the time of operation.

The acceptance of contraception after menstrual regulation is, of course, an important factor in cost-effectiveness. If no contraception is used then it is estimated that three procedures may be needed to avert a birth and in a society where lactation is common perhaps four. Estimates for births averted for contraceptive methods accepted after menstrual regulation require information on births averted by an average segment of contraceptive use in a particular locality, but this information is not readily available.

Testing for pregnancy before menstrual regulation is a justifiable expenditure if the intention is to delay the procedure for women with a negative pregnancy test, or to assist in diagnosing ectopic pregnancies. A positive pregnancy test and no evidence of products of conception in aspirated uterine contents suggest ectopic pregnancy, which may be confirmed by laparoscopy in an asymptomatic patient. Likewise, a positive pregnancy test a week after the procedure suggests continued intrauterine pregnancy or an ectopic pregnancy. The extra cost involved in delaying the procedure for women with a negative pregnancy test includes the cost of the additional visit, which may be much higher if abortion is necessary than if menstrual regulation were performed.

As might be expected, practices differ between developing and industrialized countries and, to some extent, within countries. Most menstrual regulation services in developing countries do not use either pregnancy tests or histopathological examination of uterine aspirate. These additions are often more expensive than the MR procedure itself. All procedures are performed on the first visit and a follow-up visit is generally scheduled at two weeks to check on complications and at one month if menstruation has not occurred. The patient is alerted to report to the clinic immediately in the event of heavy vaginal bleeding or abdominal pain. This is an inexpensive and cost-effective use of menstrual regulation services. It could be argued that total complications might be slightly higher than in a service where cases with negative pregnancy tests are delayed, but only *if* all or a high proportion of delayed appointments are kept – which is unlikely in many settings. It should be emphasized that if the uterine aspirate is floated on water and examined carefully with the naked eye, it is possible to see chronic villi if an intrauterine pregnancy was present. In developed countries pregnancy tests are usually performed to help eliminate possible unnecessary procedures and women with negative tests asked to return 1 week later. Some women prefer to have the procedure at the first visit, while others are willing to wait 1 week if the pregnancy test is negative.

SUMMARY

Menstrual regulation by vacuum aspiration is becoming an important post-conceptive method of fertility control. The procedure is safer and less expensive than later abortion. It has potential for wide use in both industrialized and less developed countries. Use of pregnancy tests can limit the number of unnecessary procedures, but only marginally reduce total complications. The future use of menstrual regulation will largely depend on the ready availability of the procedure.

Future research will probably turn to self-administered techniques, using, in the first instance, analogues of prostaglandin in melting vaginal suppositories. Other competing compounds that inhibit progesterone synthesis might follow. The study of long term effects of menstrual regulation by vacuum aspiration may be necessary, depending upon the outcome of similar studies in progress in first trimester abortion.

Bibliography

Dawn, C. S. and Mullick, B. (1975). Repeated menstrual regulations by suction curettage. In *Menstrual Regulation – A New Procedure for Fertility Control.* pp. 91–105 (Calcutta: Dawn Books)

Fortney, J. A., Miller, E. R. and Kessel, E. (1977). Competing risks of unnecessary procedures and complications. *Studies in Family Planning,* **8** (10), 257

Holtrop, H., Waife, R. S., Bustamante, W. and Rizo, A. (eds.) (1976). *New Developments in Fertility Regulation* (Boston: Pathfinder Fund)

Karman, H. and Potts, M. (1972). Very early abortion using a syringe as vacuum source. *Lancet,* **i,** 1051

Karim, S. M. M. (1972). Prostaglandins in fertility control. In: M. Potts and C. Ward (eds.) *New Concepts in Contraception,* p. 125 (Lancaster: MTP Press)

Kessel, E. (1975). Menstrual regulation in fertility control. In: S. Chinnatamby and N. D. W. Lionel (eds.) *Proceedings of the First International Scientific Congress of the Family Planning Association of Sri Lanka, Colombo,* January 21–26, 1974, p. 186 (Sri Lanka: Family Planning Association of Sri Lanka)

Laufe, L. E. (1977). The menstrual regulation procedure. *Studies in Family Planning,* **8** (10), 253

Loghmani, J., Mohyi, M. and Vakilzadeh, J. (1976). The use of trained nurse-midwives to perform menstrual regulation. Presented at the Annual Meeting of the Family Planning Research Association, Beverly Hills, California, 29 September to 2 October

Pion, R. M., Wabrek, A. J. and Wilson, W. B. Jr. (1972). Innovative methods in the prevention of the need for abortion. In: S. Lewit (ed.) *Abortion Techniques and Services, Proceedings of the Conference, New York, June 3–5, 1971,* pp. 14–16 (Amsterdam: Excerpta Medica)

Potter, R. G. (1972). Additional births averted when abortion is added to contraception. *Studies in Family Planning,* **3** (4), 53

Tietze, C. and Lewit, S. (1971). Legal abortions: early medical complications. *Family Planning Perspectives,* **3** (4), 6

12

The abortion epidemic

Hugo Corvalán

INTRODUCTION	201
THE CHILEAN EXPERIENCE	202
EFFECT ON FERTILITY	202
VARIATIONS IN ABORTION PATTERNS AND CONSEQUENCES	204
Morbidity and mortality	205
Cost to medical services	206
IMPLICATIONS	207
Africa	207
SOLUTIONS	208
CONCLUSIONS	211

INTRODUCTION

This chapter focuses on abortion on two levels. First, abortion as a human and public health problem and, second, and perhaps more important, the possible solution to the abortion problem. The influence of changing laws and ever-changing attitudes towards abortion has been taken into account. Information published around the world related to the subject, added to the author's personal experience in the population/family planning field in developing countries in Asia, Africa and Latin America, leads to the conclusion that, whether abortion is legal or illegal, it seems to follow a common and rather predictable pattern in relation to fertility decline.

THE CHILEAN EXPERIENCE

The analysis of abortion patterns in Chile, well documented in several works published during the 1960s, helps to illustrate what may happen to the level of abortion in a developing country which has been widely exposed to family size awareness and contraceptive usage. It is well known that fertility has declined in Chile from nearly 40/1000 in the late fifties to a reasonable 26/1000 in 1977. An impressive drop indeed, but not free of controversial and bitter discussions during the process.

It might be logical to assume that a decrease in fertility rates of this nature would be achieved by the use of methods which prevented pregnancies in the same way that a communicable disease could be prevented. Unfortunately in the Chilean case, it did not happen in this simple and ideal fashion and the marked drop in fertility rates, at least in the early days, was achieved mainly as a result of a large number of induced abortions.

EFFECT ON FERTILITY

When we study the variables affecting fertility or human reproductive behaviour then contraceptive usage and practice of abortion (legally or illegally induced) are the two variables having the most *direct* effect on fertility, although the details of their adoption will depend on the socio-cultural characteristics of the community involved. When information about contraceptives and the availability of contraceptives is absent or limited in a society which has reached a certain degree of socio-economic development and is widely exposed to propaganda about family size and contraceptive use, then induced abortion is generally used as a means of controlling family size. Contraceptives are generally first used by those groups with a higher cultural level as they have the means of acquiring information and obtaining supplies. Unfortunately, these groups are so limited in number that they do not have an important impact on fertility and/or level of abortion in the community as a whole.

According to the information on the level of contraceptive and abortion practice, obtained from surveys of women of reproductive age in Chile during the 1960s, women may be classified in three groups. Figure 1 gives a non-quantitative idea of this relationship. The group belonging to the high socio-economic and cultural level mainly use contraceptives. When induced abortion is used, it is essentially because of a failure of a contraceptive method. The women in the medium level socio-economic group are the largest users of induced abortion. This group is motivated to control family size, but does not have the initiative, the necessary information or the opportunity to resort to contraceptive means. The lower level socio-economic group has the highest fertility and makes the least use of contraception or induced abortion.

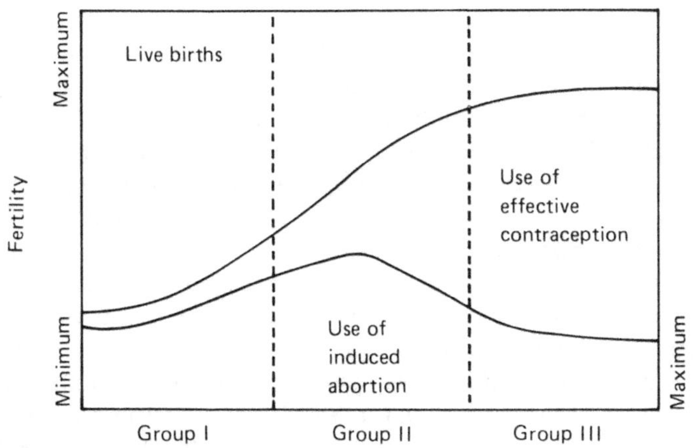

Figure 1 The relationship between abortion, fertility, contraception and socio-economic cultural level – Chile. Group I: low socio-economic level; group II: medium socio-economic level; group III: high socio-economic level

The relationship between the socio-economic cultural level and the use of induced abortion and contraceptives may be explained by the difference between those two methods. Contraception is a 'preventive' means which implies a mature and conscious attitude towards the problem. Those of us who have cared about preventive medicine know how difficult it is to practise.

The lower the cultural level is, the more a couple appear to need the recognition of an immediate problem in order to act. The individual who deals with prevention acts on probabilities and it is inherent in human nature to assume that probabilities will be favourable to one's self. Abortion, on the other hand, is a 'curative' measure that solves an already existing problem and always gives a definite result. Women are aware of the risk associated with abortion, but are prepared to accept it, just like the risk of pregnancy, with the expectation that 'it won't happen to me'. The fact that in Chile an increase in the number of induced abortions has occurred in recent decades may be explained as a displacement of induced abortion usage towards those groups of a lower socio-economic level. The medium level group who resorted to abortion at the initiation of the programme is now beginning to use contraception. The family planning programme appears to have resulted in those women who previously used abortion learning about the possibility of changing to a more rational contraceptive method and adopting it successfully. However, those women who had taken no action previously appear to have been motivated by the programme to control family size and have resorted first to the 'curative' means – abortion.

These observations give rise to controversial and sometimes bitter discussions. Some argued that the large-scale use of contraceptives has substantially decreased the already high level of illegal abortion in Chile. Others, on the contrary, argued that it was precisely the awareness about family size limitation created by the public availability of contraceptives which provoked an increase in the illegal abortion level.

Now that the heated discussions have been largely forgotten, it is possible to say that both groups were partly correct. In a small community (San Gregorio) which was used as an experimental area for a highly efficient and sophisticated family planning programme, it was shown that it is possible to replace illegal abortion (a curative practice) by a preventive one (use of modern contraception). Unfortunately experiences of this type, due to the high cost in monetary and human resources, are not possible on a national scale. Therefore, in the case of the Chilean population not exposed to an intensity of family planning programme found in San Gregorio, an increase in abortion rates of up to 25% was observed after the family planning programme was officially institutionalized (Table 1).

VARIATIONS IN ABORTION PATTERNS AND CONSEQUENCES

It is important to emphasize here that a community can react towards abortion independently of its socio-economic structure. It is possible for a lower socio-economic group to have an abortion pattern similar to a higher group, as shown in Figure 1, if a good educational and service programme is offered to them. Hence, jumping from a curative behaviour to a preventive one occurs in one step as described. However, it is important to keep in mind that in a community with a high incidence of induced abortion, a substantial decrease will not be easily achieved and this fact has been demonstrated everywhere in the developed and developing world. For instance, a study carried out in Japan by Koya shows that in the first year of a family planning programme, induced

TABLE 1 Comparison between abortion rates in San Gregorio, City and Province of Santiago after two years of family planning programme

Areas	*Abortion rates* [1] *1964*	*1966*	*Percentage of variation*	
San Gregorio	48.7*	28.7*	Reduction	41.1%*
Province of Santiago [2]	46.2	53.2	Increase	15.0%
Santiago City [3]	44.9*	56.5*	Increase	25.0%

[1] Per 1000 women of fertile age
[2] Estimation of induced abortion according to hospital statistics
[3] From Armijo and Monreal's survey in Santiago City
* Statistical confidence level – 95%

abortion increased 46% above that of the previous year. It was not until the fourth year of the programme that this rate was brought down below the pre-programme level and it took a full five years to achieve any really gratifying results. Even with a good family planning programme, it takes experience and skill to practise contraception successfully and failure rates are bound to be high until these are acquired.

Morbidity and mortality

The public health consequences of abortion vary greatly. Maternal mortality due to induced abortion is four times higher than mortality due to childbirth in those countries where methods of inducing abortion are primitive, dangerous and illegal. However, this relationship can be reversed in those societies where abortion is practised legally and in good aseptic surgical conditions. In such a situation a pregnancy may be more dangerous than an abortion induced early in gestation.

Adverse environmental conditions and dangerous methods of inducing illegal abortion in developing countries make abortion a problem of social and medical priority. It has been found, for instance in Chile, that one death occurred for every 250 women who came to the hospital for the complications of induced abortion. On the other hand, in Yugoslavia and other countries where abortion is legal and positive conditions and methods prevail, the chance of death is one in 16 000. In other words, the mortality risk of a woman undergoing an induced abortion in Chile or in other developing countries where abortion is illegal is 66.6 times the risk of a woman who has an abortion where it is legal.

The gravity of an abortion performed in a society where it is accepted legally is quite different when compared with a country where it is illegal and therefore subject to prosecution. It is easy to neglect other aspects of induced abortion when measuring the magnitude of abortion by mortality or gynaecological morbidity. For example, the probable psychic reaction in women, personal and financial cost, even risking abandoned children and broken families, can be significant. Of even greater importance than mortality is the continuance of morbidity due to illegally induced abortion. The major cause of this morbidity is uterine and tubal infection which results in post-abortion infertility. These infections can be controlled provided adequate measures and resources are available.

Cost to medical services

Another important factor to be considered in abortion as a public health problem, besides maternal mortality, is its implication for national health systems. It has been reported in the statistics of some developing countries that complicated abortions put a heavy burden on the already insufficient medical care services. In countries where illegal abortion is already an epidemic, or is rapidly becoming one, the proportion of complicated abortions compared with normal deliveries is surprisingly high. Therefore, the hospitals are severely affected in their ability to provide obstetric care, as approximately one third of the resources are diverted to the management of complicated abortions.

In most instances, the interface where the medical care services first deal with the complicated abortion is the emergency service. There is, accordingly, a justified interest in studying the amount of resources directed through emergency services to deal with this morbidity. It has been reported that in some places, complicated abortions accounted for 42% of all consultations, i.e. the most important category among emergency admissions. Furthermore, 18% of bed-days were absorbed by complicated abortions, competing very seriously with acute medical and surgical episodes requiring emergency admission and treatment. Seventeen per cent of the total blood transfusions were administered to abortion patients; in terms of volume of blood this accounted for 27% of the always scarce blood of transfusion services.

These hospital statistics represent only a partial picture of what may happen in the community as a whole. Surveys in urban settlements show that up to 50% of women interviewed volunteered a history of abortion of some kind and nearly 30% gave a definite history of one or more induced abortions. Furthermore, it has been found that there is a tendency for certain groups of women to resort to abortion repeatedly. In the above mentioned surveys a quarter of the women accounted for 60% of all abortions. The recognition of the existence of these groups may have practical implications for preventive measures as we will discuss later.

IMPLICATIONS

The facts described above are from Latin American countries where abortion reached an epidemic character during recent years. However, it is the author's opinion that other continents have still to face the major part of the abortion problem. Abortion in most Asian and African countries has not yet reached an epidemic level, mainly due to their stage of socio-economic development. However, it can be foreseen with some accuracy, that many African and Asian countries will be confronted with an abortion problem similar in magnitude and gravity to that faced by many contemporary Latin American countries.

Government and private organizations in Africa and Asia are developing different contraceptive distribution projects, with the backing of motivational and educational campaigns at every level. The degree of success of these schemes varies from country to country, but undoubtedly awareness about spacing pregnancies and limiting family size has been created. My assumption is that, as a result of increased awareness of family planning and as a result of socio-economic development created by governmental actions, abortions are going to become an increasingly significant problem in many areas in Africa and Asia, not to mention those of the remaining Latin American countries which were not affected by the 'abortion epidemic' during the nineteen sixties and early seventies. The consequences of such an epidemic, both in health and social terms, are easy to foresee. Moreover, the technology to prevent and/or treat abortions, therefore avoiding the extra cost to the health structure in these countries, is available at our fingertips.

Africa

In an interim report recently prepared by Dr Monreal and presented at the Workshop on the Strategy for Abortion Management in Africa (organized by the IPPF Africa Regional Office) it is reported that illegal abortion is present in most African countries, or at least in the capital cities. The incidence is still low, but there is no doubt that sooner or later it will increase. In some cities it was found that there were three deaths out of every 300 patients hospitalized for abortion. Compared with other areas of the world this figure represents a very high mortality rate for illegal abortions.

Most of these deaths were the result of dangerous methods in the hands of irresponsible persons, causing perforation of the uterus and other serious septic complications which can result in death. It is more because of this high mortality than because of the high incidence, that illegal abortion already represents a major public health problem in African urban areas. The situation will tend to get worse. The increased demand for education and employment opportunities will accelerate the existing process of immigration to capital cities and other urban areas. Women will also demand a different status, equal rights and an end to sex discrimination. The process of social and cultural changes will continue. The idea of large families and the association of women and fertility will change and, among other consequences, both incidence and severity of illegal abortions will increase.

It is the responsibility of governments and non-governmental organizations to anticipate an increase in the number of abortions and take appropriate action. Currently, there are several schemes for organizing sex education projects, innovative means of reaching communities with effective contraceptives and liberalization of restrictive laws related to contraceptive use and surgical methods of family planning. However, ideally, in the areas affected by a large number of complicated abortions and the areas likely to be affected in the near future, comprehensive programmes of fertility control should be set up. Use of all the available techniques must be emphasized. For instance, preventive measures such as well-orientated population education and sex education campaigns should be integrated with modern contraceptive delivery services. Early diagnosis of pregnancy should also play an important role, especially in those areas where current laws would permit early pregnancy termination.

These measures coupled with efficient post-partum and post-abortion contraception and sterilization should be able to prevent a large number of unwanted pregnancies and consequently induced abortions. It is important to recall the existence of groups of women who will resort to abortion repeatedly to control their fertility. The identification of such groups is of paramount importance in any rational abortion control programme.

SOLUTIONS

There are several ways of cutting down or eliminating abortion as a burden to national health structures, although many of them may be considered unorthodox. In order to provide an example of these potential measures, I will mention a personal experience of only anecdotal value, but which illustrates the point. A young general practitioner (friend of mine) working in a semi-urban community was in charge of a small hospital which was facing a heavy case load of abortion patients. Complications resulting from induced abortions accounted for more than 70% of occupied beds in the obstetric ward. Even knowing that such an initiative was beyond current legal codes, the physician assembled the well-known group of abortionists and quack doctors belonging to the community and taught them the basic techniques of asepsis and curettage and the safe and rational use of antibiotics. He also trained them in the use of modern contraceptives.

After several weeks of this unorthodox 'training' the admission for complicated abortions fell dramatically in a steady downward trend over time. This way of tackling the problem will not necessarily decrease the actual number of abortions performed in a community, unless a sharp increase in the use of postabortion contraception takes place. However, in practical terms, there is a significant saving in health costs as the number of complicated induced abortions fall and fewer hospital beds are occupied by these patients. In other words, it is necessary to recognize that unless exceptional preventive measures are taken, it can be difficult in the short term to really control the total number of induced abortions. Faced with this reality, it is only logical and humane to provide the means and resources that enable those groups with limited access to private physicians to solve their problem. Once an unwanted pregnancy has occurred, it is almost inevitable that it will end in an induced abortion – even where abortion is illegal.

Personally, I have treated many women for complications occurring as a result of attempted illegal abortion by the most crude and dangerous means, such as the inserting of knitting needles in the uterus. When these women were told that because of the legal situation in the country their pregnancy should continue, their invariable reply was that next time they would be more thorough when attempting to destroy the fetus. And in most cases they certainly were and I had to treat them for infected incomplete abortion, anaemia and other severe complications.

Exploring existing laws and analysing the possibilities which exist within this framework for early pregnancy termination is a second alternative worth exploring and one which may lead to an amelioration of the abortion problem without upsetting the medical or political establishment. Thirdly, the prompt treatment of incomplete abortion, whether induced or spontaneous, must be obligatory in any obstetric–gynaecological out-patient service. Nowhere in the world does the prompt treatment of abortion conflict with laws, however restrictive. Therefore, there can be no excuse for delaying the availability of such services. The role of vacuum aspiration and the opportunity for post-abortal contraceptive advice is significant and must be utilized.

The examples described above clarify the existence of sound alternatives which can be easily used anywhere in the world by those who wish to apply themselves to the solution of the abortion problem, without getting tangled in the manipulation and/or interpretation of restrictive laws. A human solution for the millions of women affected by the very human problem of unwanted pregnancy is urgently required.

A rather different approach towards the solution of illegally induced abortions is the concentration of efforts and resources in changing restrictive laws in those countries already affected by the abortion epidemic and especially in those countries on the threshold of becoming affected. The main purpose of liberalization of abortion laws is to make the procedure available safely by taking abortion away from the quack doctors and the hidden abortionist, and therefore reducing the risks involved in clandestine operations. As emphasized before, illegal abortions constitute an exceedingly high risk for the woman with an unwanted pregnancy. In addition, by bringing women with unwanted pregnancies into legal, public services, it is more likely that they will also be brought into contact with realistic contraceptive services.

From this perspective, legalized abortions would also achieve an improvement in two other pressing areas of concern. One is in reducing the pressure on the health system resources from complicated abortions and the other is related to the concept of social justice. It must not be forgotten that those who suffer most under restricted laws regulating abortion are the low income groups which cannot afford to pay the professional doctors' fees for a safe, if illegal, abortion and who are therefore segregated from the safe and adequate termination of a pregnancy. Moreover, it is within the lower strata of society that one finds the high-risk groups, i.e. women who for well-known reasons have not had access to contraception and resort to abortion under the worst possible conditions.

Yet, considered as a public health tool and a measure of preventive medicine, legal abortions are not entirely free from potential shortcomings:

* abortion contravenes the values and religious morals of a proportion of the population in many countries. This can be expected to create opposition, or at least lack of enthusiasm, for liberal abortion legislation;
* a legalization of abortion could give rise to prejudice against the family planning programmes and, perhaps, against contraception in general. There are valid reasons for wondering if some people will tend to seek solutions for a problem once it has become evident, rather than try to prevent such a crisis happening;
* even legal abortions require medical manpower and facilities, both of

which are scarce, so that there is again a danger that quacks will pre-empt the field;

* finally, legal abortion performed under good conditions is not entirely free of complications.

Under these circumstances, we strongly advocate that before any decision is taken concerning legalization of abortion, a careful appraisal of the implications and foreseeable consequences of such a policy can and should be made. This is even more important in those developing countries where health resources are limited. Any decision concerning liberal abortion legislation should be taken as part of a comprehensive preventive plan and not, as is often the case, as an isolated measure without the proper theoretical framework for operation. Moreover, additional research in the area of abortion is urgently needed in order to provide some of the answers required for a definition of such policies, based on satisfactory and reliable evidence. Great attention and priority should be given to Africa and Asia where limited experience exists so far.

CONCLUSIONS

To sum up, we first advocate strong preventive measures to arrest abortion epidemics. The rational use of community education is essential to provide information on the hazards involved in illegal abortion and the rewards obtainable through planned parenthood in terms of health and well-being. The knowledge on abortion generated by academic institutions is, unfortunately, very often kept from the general public. It is necessary to provide the channels for this knowledge to reach the community and the interface of the health services where it can be applied in the daily work.

Sex education should not be ignored and every effort should be made in trying to introduce it as early as possible in a child's life through formal and non-formal education. It is of great importance, in any preventive control programme, to provide detailed and personal education to all contraceptive consumers with emphasis on problems relating to abortion. This educational component of the programme must include the potential 'client' and, ideally, should be incorporated in the follow-up of the women using contraception, as well as their husbands. Here again, one should bear in mind that activities must devote special attention to women at a high risk of having repeated abortions.

The training of manpower for the proposed control programme is essential and should be designed to fulfil the needs and demands of the varied and broad range of consumers' attitudes, which the programme is likely to encounter.

On the one hand, the programme can be expected to promote a high degree of satisfaction and confidence on the part of the population it is serving. On the other, this confidence is essential to avoid failures in the use of contraceptive methods as a high proportion of these failures will subsequently turn to induced abortion.

We would like here to introduce a word about family planning services and their relevance as part of a preventive scheme to check abortion numbers. If one looks at the whole picture of contraceptive services provided around the developing world, it is evident that there are appreciable differences. There are clinics dealing with only one method of contraception, whereas others offer every modern and acceptable traditional method. Some places restrict their services to women with certain precisely defined qualifications while other clinics are open to any woman wishing to control her fertility. It is of paramount importance for the success of the preventive programme for it to be established firmly on the basis of sound criteria in the regulation of its services.

First, surgical sterilization should be part and parcel of the preventive programme. It seems unreasonable to force young women who have reached a desired family size to continue using contraception – with the several small side-effects that may occur and with an ever present though small risk of failure – for the rest of their reproductive life. It is only humane to offer a terminal method for fertility control. With advances in technology, it is well known that voluntary sterilization requires limited manpower and financial resources and can be performed in out-patient clinics (see also Chapter 10). I consider an abortion prevention programme without sterilization to be crippled.

Second, it must be recognized that the use of modern contraception requires certain skills and that, especially at the beginning of contraceptive use, failures are bound to happen. It is also known that the most effective method, even properly used, carries a risk of failure.

I consider it a moral responsibility for those running the programme to advise users and potential users of the failure risks involved and would like to suggest that their responsibility should extend a little beyond the mere information. I feel it would be only fair to offer the clients and potential programme clients a solution in cases where they have become accidentally pregnant whilst using a contraceptive. Obviously, for many women the solution is an early pregnancy termination, which could be performed in an out-patient clinic using menstrual regulation kits (see Chapter 11) or vacuum aspiration. Either or both could be manipulated by trained paramedical personnel under the supervision of doctors and at a very low cost.

The solutions of the current abortion epidemic and of the epidemic that can be seen arising in some countries and continents are not technically complicated. They are readily available to any country that wishes to tackle the problem. Some of the solutions proposed here are controversial and others may be difficult to accept for different cultural, moral or political reasons. However, any governments or non-governmental organizations that decide and are willing to solve the abortion problem must face the fact that currently there are no other technical solutions. They will probably have to choose a mix of the different approaches discussed here. The common denominator is always the dual attempt to prevent pregnancies – realizing that some degree of failure is inevitable – and the interruption of unwanted pregnancies when they occur. The abortion road has only one end and solution – and this solution is, or at least should be, in the hands of the affected woman. Society should facilitate her decision.

Bibliography

Armijo, R. and Monreal, T. (1965). The problem of induced abortion in Chile. *Milbank Memorial Fund Quarterly*, **43**, 263

Corvalan, H. (1972). Induced abortion as a public health problem in Chile, MSc Medical Demography degree thesis, London School of Hygiene and Tropical Medicine (mimeo).

David, H. (ed.) (1974). *Abortion Research: International Experience*. (Massachusetts: Lexington Books)

Faundes, A., Rodriguez, R. and Avendaño, O. (1969). *El Programa de Planificación Familiar de San Gregorio*. (mimeo)

Koya, Y. (1966). *Harmful Effects of Induced Abortion*. (Family Planning Federation of Japan)

Monreal, Γ. and Armijo, R. (1968). Evaluation of the programme for the prevention of induced abortion and for family planning in the City of Santiago. *Revista Médica de Chile*, **96**, 605

Monreal T. (1978). Illegal abortion in selected African capital cities. Paper presented at the workshop on the strategy for abortion management in Africa. (In press)

Moore, E. (1971). *Inventory of Information on Induced Abortion*. (New York: Columbia University, International Institute for the Study of Human Reproduction)

Omran, A. R. (ed.) (1976). *Liberalization of Abortion Laws: Implications*. (Chapel Hill, North Carolina: Carolina Population Center)

Potter, R. G. (1972). Additional births averted when abortion is added to contraception. *Studies in Family Planning*, **3**, 53

Potts, M., Diggory, P. C. and Peel, J. (1977). *Abortion*. (Cambridge: Cambridge University Press)

Raquena, M. (1965). Social and economic correlates of induced abortion in Chile. *Demography*, **2**, 33

Raquena, M. (1968). The problem of induced abortion in Latin America. *Demography*, **5**, 785

Raquena, M. and Monreal, T. (1968). Evaluation of induced abortion control and family planning in Chile. *Milbank Memorial Fund Quarterly*, **46** (3), 191

van der Tak, J. (1974). *Abortion, Fertility and Changing Legislation: An International Review*. (Massachusetts: Lexington Books)

Viel, B. (1976). *The Demographic Explosion; The Latin American Experience.* (New York: Irvington Publishers)

Note. The ideas expressed in this chapter are those of the author, and do not necessarily represent those of the United Nations Fund for Population Activities.

13

Future developments in fertility control

Roger Short

HUMAN SEXUALITY	215
NATURAL METHODS OF FERTILITY REGULATION	217
TOWARDS A HEALTHIER STATE OF INFERTILITY	218
The uterus and the ovaries	218
The breasts	220
FUTURE CONTRACEPTIVE DEVELOPMENT	222

HUMAN SEXUALITY

Before we can start to consider realistically the probable success of any future fertility control techniques, we must begin by taking a general look at ourselves as a species, and the role of sexuality in our lives. It is man's intellectual failing that he is fascinated by minutiae and detail, whereas forward planning can only be based on the simplest of concepts and the broadest of generalizations. In a few hundred words, how could we summarize what is known of our reproductive behaviour?

Surely the unique feature of man which distinguishes him from all other mammals is that he has used his sexuality for recreation and not just for procreation. The suppression of oestrus in women, whereby they can seek and obtain gratification from sexual intercourse on any day of their lives, from puberty to old age, has meant that human sexuality has become a most important social bonding force between man and woman. Indeed, it seems that primitive man was initially unaware of any direct relationship between intercourse and conception. This is quite understandable when one remembers that a girl began having intercourse at puberty, when she developed the physical attributes that made her attractive to men, but she would probably not conceive for several years thereafter because the initial menstrual cycles are usually anovulatory. Under such circumstances, it would have been impossible to deduce that intercourse led to pregnancy. It was only when man began to domesticate animals that the facts of life dawned on him; animals only copulate when the female is in oestrus and there is a high probability that the female will conceive at that time, and give birth at a predictable moment thereafter. Even today, it is only with the wisdom of hindsight that man can guess which act of intercourse might have resulted in conception and the probability of doing so will be less than 1% in any case. If man, uniquely, has developed his sexuality for other than reproductive purposes and if sex has really become the social cement of the pair-bond, no contraceptive technique that interferes with the act or the emotion of intercourse can ever be totally acceptable in the long term. And we must think in the long term, because having progressively eliminated those natural checks and balances that hitherto kept our rate of population growth in equilibrium with our environment (checks such as late age at puberty, high neonatal mortality rate, and a long birth interval resulting from lactational amenorrhoea) we are going to be increasingly dependent on artificial forms of contraception forever more.

Another factor that we should consider is the nature of the pair-bond. Mammals show three basic patterns of mating behaviour: monogamy, which is rather rare; promiscuity, which is even rarer; and polygyny, a form of polygamy, in which one male mates successfully with more than one female. Polygyny is by far the commonest mammalian strategy and although it may be contrary to the Western, Christian ethic, several lines of evidence suggest that man is indeed a polygynous species. For example, detailed anthropological investigations of 185 contemporary 'primitive' human societies showed that only 16% were exclusively monogamous, whereas in all the others polygynous marriages were permitted, although economic considerations and a shortage of women meant that in practice monogamy occurred in half of them. It may be that serial monogamy represents the human norm, being a compromise between our polygynous natures and the need to maintain the parental pair-bond for the benefit of the children. Our polygyny even shows up in the mirror; the fact that men are appreciably taller and heavier than women is an example of enhanced male sexual selection made possible by polygyny.

Given these polygynous tendencies, it seems likely that factors such as the rising divorce rate in Western society, so often condemned as moral decadence, is merely man reverting to type. As we relax the constraints hitherto imposed by rigorous adherence to the Christian ethic, we can expect the divorce rate to continue to rise, and a change of marital partners may become the normal pattern of behaviour for many. If this prediction proves correct, it may well alter our attitudes to the acceptability of ultimate forms of contraception, such as irreversible male and female sterilization.

NATURAL METHODS OF FERTILITY REGULATION

It is also profitable to spend a few moments considering the way in which Nature regulates fertility, and how man has attempted to follow her example. Since the female eutherian mammal lactates, whereas her male partner cannot, and since she also has to nurture the growing embryo in her uterus for a relatively long period of time, it follows that her energy investment in producing a new generation is much, much greater than the male's. She is the limiting resource, and therefore Nature has not unnaturally selected the female rather than the male for fertility regulation. Thus, it seems sensible that we, too, should devote most of our research effort to developing female rather than male forms of contraception, despite the apparent male chauvinism of such an approach.

Demographically the most important factor regulating female reproduction is the time interval between successive births, and most mammals have made use of lactation to inhibit a return to fertility after birth. We are still exploring the ways in which this inhibitory effect is brought about, but present evidence would suggest that the inhibition is initially caused by a train of afferent impulses from the nipple to the brain, produced by the suckling action of the infant. Anything that reduces suckling frequency can therefore be expected to enhance fertility. These afferent impulses seem to act at two levels. There is a central effect, which alters hypothalamic sensitivity to steroidal feedback, making the hypothalamus revert to its pre-pubertal condition of being insensitive to the positive feedback effects of gonadal steroids. In addition, there is a peripheral effect, probably mediated by prolactin, which alters gonadal responsiveness to pituitary gonadotrophins. If these do indeed represent Nature's mechanisms for the regulation of fertility, it is humbling to realize that we have not yet been able to emulate either of them.

TOWARDS A HEALTHIER STATE OF INFERTILITY

The way in which contraceptive development has proceeded so far has been both illogical and irrational. We have sought in desperation for anything that worked. The advent of new techniques such as the pill and the intrauterine device have stemmed the flood of births in many areas of the world and have given us a breathing space. We must now use this precious time to develop a contraceptive strategy for the future. Sex is fun and always has been. We cannot expect any but the most dedicated to adopt a self-denying form of contraception like Malthusian total abstinence, or the periodic abstinence of the rhythm method. Since reproductive success is essential for the survival of the species, tremendous selection pressure has been brought to bear in the past to maximise our fertility. We are therefore ill-adapted to our new lifestyle of prolonged periods of enforced infertility. We must ask ourselves some critical questions: what is the optimal state of repose for a uterus that we no longer need to produce babies, an ovary that is no longer required to ovulate, and a breast that we do not want to produce milk? Only when we have answered these questions will we be in a position to offer women what they deserve, namely healthy infertility.

The uterus and the ovaries

As far as the uterus is concerned, we do not really know the answer, but we can make a few guesses. In the first place, an endless succession of menstrual cycles represents a self-induced disorder of civilized communities practising contraception. Menstruation must have been a relatively infrequent event for our primitive hunter-gatherer ancestors, who spent the greater part of their reproductive lives in lactational amenorrhoea, interspersed with four or five pregnancies. In Western society, we know that 10% of women lose more than 100 ml of blood a month during menstruation, and whilst this may be inconsequential for them, a comparable loss might represent a severe metabolic demand for a woman in a developing country on a marginal plane of nutrition, starved of protein, and already anaemic as a result of intercurrent hookworm and malaria. To this must be added the social, religious and emotional inconvenience of menstruation, and the cost of sanitary protection. In theory at least, there would thus be much to commend the development of forms of contraception that decreased the frequency and/or the severity of menstruation. We already have proof that this would be highly acceptable to educated women in a developed country, and it might also prove acceptable to Hindu, Muslim and Buddhist women, all of whom are subjected to socially restrictive taboos during menstruation. Whether it would find favour with the great mass of poorly educated women in developing countries is more problematical. It seems likely that any woman might well resent prolonged amenorrhoea in the period prior to her first pregnancy, since she would rightly regard it as a potential threat to her future fertility. However, many women might welcome a prolongation of the normal period of postpartum amenorrhoea, so that they could achieve adequate spacing between successive births. Certainly amenorrhoea would be even more acceptable to those who had completed their families and did not wish to conceive again.

Unfortunately, we know ali too little about the basic physiology of menstruation to enable us to develop new techniques for producing oligo- or amenorrhoea. We have known since the 1930s that the basic cause of menstruation was sloughing of the secretory endometrium, resulting from spasm of the spiral arterioles which is produced by a withdrawal of oestrogen and/or progesterone. More recently, we have come to realize that prostaglandins are involved in the process, although it is still not clear whether they play a causal or a consequential role. Certainly the systematic administration of prostaglandin synthetase inhibitors like indomethacin, fluphenamic acid or mephenamic acid reduces the pain and severity of menstrual blood loss.

Were it not for the existence of menstruation, contraceptive development would be a much simpler problem to solve. Women will tolerate quite heavy menstrual blood loss provided that its timing is predictable so that they can take appropriate precautions beforehand. But sudden, unexpected 'breakthrough bleeding' or even mild 'spotting' is most undesirable, and it is this that has so bedevilled attempts to develop acceptable long-acting steroidal injections or implants as forms of contraception.

Sex hormones can be divided into three categories depending on their biological effects – androgens, oestrogens and progestagens. Androgens cannot be used for female contraception due to masculinizing effects. Oestrogens are undoubtedly the most potent inhibitors of gonadotrophin secretion and hence of ovulation, but on their own they produce unpleasant side-effects such as nausea, and long-term treatment poses a carcinogenic hazard, particularly for the endometrium. Progestagens have far fewer known adverse side-effects, but are also much less efficient at inhibiting gonadotrophin secretion and preventing ovulation. If used on their own, even in large doses, it seems that some residual follicular activity persists in the ovaries, and the waxing and waning of this ovarian oestrogen secretion, as follicles develop and then become atretic, allows the development of a secretory endometrium, which periodically sloughs following oestrogen withdrawal and produces the unexpected 'breakthrough bleed'. This can be overcome by giving massive doses of progestagens which will ultimately inhibit all follicular development in the ovaries and produce an atrophic endometrium which cannot slough and bleed. The drawback here, however, is that the pituitary inhibition is now so profound that it may take many months or even years to restore normal ovarian function following cessation of the contraceptive therapy.

If one uses a combined treatment with a progestagen and an oestrogen, it is possible to obtain a synergistic effect with relatively low doses of both hormones. Centrally, this combined treatment effectively inhibits gonadotrophin secretion and prevents ovulation, whilst peripherally it maintains a secretory endometrium, thereby minimizing the risk of endometrial carcinoma and preventing unexpected breakthrough bleeding. If the combined steroid therapy is kept up, this secretory endometrium can be maintained for prolonged periods of time, and a withdrawal bleed will follow cessation of the therapy.

And so we are faced with the dilemma of the endometrium. It seems unwise to use oestrogen alone as a contraceptive, since this will produce a proliferative type of endometrium which is susceptible to neoplastic change. Use of a combined oestrogen/progestagen mixture produces a secretory endometrium, controls menstruation and reduces the cancer risk, but we have no idea how long this secretory state can or should be maintained. Use of a progestagen alone gives a poor control of pituitary activity and the resultant waxing and waning of ovarian oestrogen secretion results in the production of a secretory endometrium with periodic undesirable breakthrough bleeds. In order to produce an atrophic endometrium comparable to that seen in women during lactational amenorrhoea, it is necessary to use such large doses of progestagen that it may take some time to restore normal ovarian activity after one has ceased taking the contraceptive. Perhaps steroid therapy is not the best way of achieving a healthy, resting uterus.

The breasts

When thinking about contraceptive development, little or no thought has been given to the breast. And yet the mammary gland is an integral part of the reproductive tract, profoundly influenced by sex hormones, and a constant supply of breast milk is still the staple diet for most of the newborn children of the world. The breast's susceptibility to hormones is probably reflected in the high incidence of breast cancer, with a lifetime incidence of one woman in 20 in developed countries – and this figure may still be on the increase; fortunately, there is as yet a much lower incidence rate in developing countries. We know that the incidence can be reduced by factors such as a late age at menarche, an early age at first pregnancy, and an early natural or artificial menopause. This epidemiological evidence, together with much direct experimental evidence from animals, strongly suggests that oestrogen is involved in the aetiology of the condition, and it is a plausible working hypothesis to suggest that the breast, like the uterus, is ill-adapted to prolonged periods of infertility.

The human breast is unique amongst all primates in that it undergoes full anatomical development at puberty, whereas in monkeys mammary enlargement only occurs towards the end of the first pregnancy. This pubertal development in the human is due primarily to stromal hypertrophy and since breast enlargement is the first clinical sign of impending puberty, occurring long before the first ovulation, it must mean that the stromal tissue of the human breast has become exquisitely oestrogen-sensitive. We know that the breast undergoes considerable volume changes during the menstrual cycle, collapsing at the time of menstruation, and it may be that it is ill-adapted to cope with such monthly cycles of hypertrophy and regression, particularly if it has not been transformed into a fully functional, lactating organ beforehand.

So what does all this mean for contraceptive development? Firstly, it becomes extremely important to determine whether progesterone exerts a 'sparing effect', protecting the gland against oestrogenic stimulation. There is some evidence to suggest that progesterone may interfere with oestrogen receptor activity in target organs; if this is the case, we might expect to find that menstrual cycles induced by the combined oral contraceptive pill are less likely to give rise to breast cancer than normal menstrual cycles in which the gland will be exposed to unopposed oestrogenic stimulation for the first half of the cycle. So far, all the large-scale epidemiological surveys of oral contraceptive users are in agreement that the Pill does not seem to increase the incidence of breast cancer and probably lowers the incidence of benign lesions and cysts in the breast. Since people who have had a benign breast lesion are more likely to develop a breast malignancy subsequently, there is some hope that as more and more Pill takers enter the high breast cancer risk age group, we may find that the Pill has actually lowered the incidence of breast cancer. But it will be particularly interesting to see if Pill-taking in those 'sensitizing' years between menarche and the first pregnancy has a protective effect, because the epidemiological evidence points strongly to this as the critical time when pre-cancerous changes may be initiated.

Little thought has been given in the developed world to the effects of contraceptive steroids on established lactation, and yet any interference with the food supply of the infant could have disastrous effects in the developing world, where breast feeding is still the norm, and should be encouraged to remain so. There is evidence that the combined oral contraceptive, particularly with relatedly high oestrogen content, may diminish the milk yield, whereas the progestagen-only minipill seems to have no deleterious effect. However, these are empirical observations and the precise mechanism by which these effects are brought about have still to be determined. One clue might come from the recent discovery that the tactile sensitivity of the breast, and in particular of the nipple, is under hormonal control. The breast is apparently 'anaesthetized' by the high steroid levels in late pregnancy, to such an extent that nipple stimulation will not evoke a reflex prolactin discharge. However, within 24 hours of parturition the nipple becomes extremely sensitive, so that the suckling stimulus results in a reflex prolactin release, thereby ensuring a continued supply of milk for the future. It seems likely that oral contraceptives interfere with the tactile sensitivity of the breast postpartum in the same way that they have been shown to do during the cycle: this would therefore decrease the prolactin discharge and ultimately curtail milk production. Oral contraceptives may also interfere centrally, exerting a direct inhibitory effect on prolactin secretion at the level of the hypothalamus or pituitary. If we are to develop contraceptives that are tailor-made for the lactating woman, we need to take these factors into account.

I think I have said enough about ways in which we might try to achieve this goal of 'healthy infertility' in the future. We need to adopt a more positive attitude to contraception, emphasizing that it could be used to minimize the health risks of our enforced state of infertility; at the moment, we have an essentially negative attitude, regarding the risks of contraception as the inevitable price we must pay for restricting our fertility.

FUTURE CONTRACEPTIVE DEVELOPMENT

What chance is there of seeing any of these theories translated into practice in the foreseeable future? A glance at each annual report of the World Health Organisation Special Programme of Research, Development and Research Training in Human Reproduction is a fascinating window into the world of contraceptive development. In spite of the availability of motivation, money and manpower, one has to admit that progress has been painfully slow. It is doubtful if any major new approach to contraception will be commercially available before the end of this century.

Attempts to develop male contraceptives have been bedevilled by the fact that compounds that inhibit the spermatogenic activity of the testis also inhibit its androgen production, and rightly or wrongly men think that their androgen levels are necessary for their libido, aggression, drive, machismo and all those other characteristics that make us so objectionable – and so fascinating! We do not have really adequate forms of androgen replacement therapy, and although some androgen and progestagen mixtures have been in clinical trials and are capable of inhibiting pituitary activity sufficiently to produce a degree of oligospermia, we do not know how oligospermic a man must become before he can be considered infertile. There is the additional drawback that there is a time lag of 2 or 3 months between starting the treatment and the development of the oligospermia. Thus it seems unlikely that we will have an acceptable steroidal injection, implant or pill for men in the near future.

At one time it was hoped that these difficulties could be overcome by selectively inhibiting the testes' spermatogenic function, whilst leaving their androgenic activity unimpaired; there is evidence that Nature might be able to do just this by means of a hormone, inhibin, produced by the Sertoli cells and acting on the pituitary to depress FSH secretion and hence regulate the spermatogenic process. But the more we discover about inhibin, the less likely it seems that it will be clinically useful as a male contraceptive. Another approach that still holds some promise is the development of non-toxic chemical compounds that interfere with the metabolism and fertilizing capacity of formed spermatozoa. Professor Waites has recently shown that a group of simple, non-toxic, chlorinated sugars being developed as artificial sweeteners can rapidly induce infertility in male rats, and fertility can be rapidly restored once the treatment is stopped. But even if such compounds were to prove effective in man, it would still be 10–15 years before they became generally available, such is the stringency of the animal toxicity testing and human clinical trial procedures that must now be adopted before any new compound can be brought onto the open market.

Another area that has excited much attention amongst research workers has been the immunological control of fertility. Although the simple approach of immunizing the female against the spermatozoa of the male has not proved an effective contraceptive technique, at least in animal studies, immunization of the female against specific hormones or substances seems more encouraging. For example, we know that the human placenta secretes chorionic gonadotrophin (HCG) from about the time of implantation, and that this acts on the corpus luteum in the mother's ovary, preventing its regression and thus maintaining the supply of hormones necessary for implantation and early embryonic development. Chorionic gonadotrophin is made up of two subunits – an α subunit which is shared in common with Follicle Stimulating Hormone (FSH), Luteinizing Hormone (LH) and Thyroid Stimulating Hormone (TSH) from the anterior pituitary gland, and a β subunit which is hormone specific. If one immunizes monkeys against the β subunit of the human hormone, they produce antibodies against it and are then incapable of maintaining a pregnancy, although they continue to ovulate, and fertilization occurs normally.

Unfortunately, as the antibody titres begin to wane after 1–2 years, the monkeys start to have abortions at later and later stages of pregnancy until ultimately their fertility is restored and they give birth to normal, full-term live offspring. If these late abortions occurred in women, particularly in developing countries following such an immunization procedure, they might prove fatal. Nevertheless, work is still progressing along these lines, notably in India, the United States and Australia, aimed at modifying the human β subunit to make it more antigenic in women. Limited clinical trials of the immunization procedure have even been initiated in certain countries.

Yet another immunological approach has been to raise antibodies against the small decapeptide hormone, Gonadotrophin Releasing Hormone (GnRH), which is produced in the hypothalamus and which controls the pituitary secretion of FSH and LH. Immunization of male or female laboratory animals successfully inhibits pituitary gonadotrophin secretion; the testes of the males regress and spermatogenesis ceases, but unfortunately the androgen levels also fall. In the female, ovulation ceases, although there is still some residual follicular development in the ovaries. It may be that this is more akin to the state of the ovaries in lactational amenorrhoea and if it is true that human female libido, in contrast to male libido, is relatively independent of sex hormone levels, then such a state of ovarian (and uterine) quiescence would at least be theoretically acceptable as a form of contraception. But maybe immunization is not the best way to produce it. Recently it has been shown that another way of blocking the gonadal response to FSH and LH is to give excessively large amounts of the hypothalamic releasing hormone or one of its more potent synthetic analogues. These can be administered intranasally as snuff and appears to be totally devoid of any adverse side-effects. The only obvious snag here is that the common cold would have a pronounced anticontraceptive effect! The intranasal route of administration may also be useful for steroid hormones, since preliminary evidence in monkeys suggests that extremely small amounts of conventional oral contraceptives can be given by nasal spray, thereby in some unknown way inhibiting pituitary gonadotrophin secretion without elevating systemic blood levels or having effects on peripheral target organs such as the uterus.

We cannot leave the subject of future fertility control techniques without some mention of abortion. Although it would be foolish to imagine that abortion will ultimately be adopted as a primary method of contraception, it is equally foolish to expect any contraceptive programme to operate successfully without backup abortion facilities. Vacuum aspiration of the uterus can be performed as an outpatient procedure for first-trimester abortions and it is remarkably effective, safe and relatively painless. It seems unlikely and undesirable that self-administered once-a-month 'menstrual induction' will be adopted as a form of contraception by any but the most ardent and affluent women's libbers. But if we could develop self-administered medical as opposed to surgical procedures for first-trimester abortion, these would have much to commend them both in developing and developed countries. Early hopes that the prostaglandins might fulfil this role by virtue of the luteolytic action that they are known to have in animals have not been realized; unfortunately, they do not seem to be luteolytic in women and when given in large doses produce painful gastrointestinal side-effects. However, some of the new synthetic prostaglandin analogues are beginning to vie with vacuum aspiration as a safe and effective way of inducing first-trimester abortions and are already the method of choice for second trimester abortions. Perhaps new compounds will be developed that are effective early abortifacients which can be taken by mouth; they would certainly be in great demand.

If we are realistic, we must admit that the main changes in contraceptive usage during the rest of this century are more likely to be improvements of existing techniques – a combined oral contraceptive pill with a lower incidence of side effects, an intra-uterine device that is more effective and does not increase menstrual blood loss – rather than in the development of radically new techniques. And at the end of the day, we must not be so blinded by sophistication that we forget the simplest of methods; after all, nobody has yet been killed by a condom.

Bibliography

Ford, W. C. L. and Waites, G. M. H. (1978). A reversible contraceptive action of some 6-chloro-6-deoxy sugars in the male rat. *Journal of Reproduction and Fertility*, **52**, 153

Loudon, N. B., Foxwell, M., Potts, D. M., Guild, A. L. and Short, R. V. (1977). Acceptability of an oral contraceptive that reduces the frequency of menstruation: the tri-cycle pill regimen. *British Medical Journal*, **2**, 487

Milligan, D., Drife, J. O. and Short, R. V. (1975). Changes in breast volume during normal menstrual cycle and after oral contraceptives. *British Medical Journal*, **4**, 494

Robinson, J. E. and Short, R. V. (1977). Changes in breast sensitivity at puberty, during the menstrual cycle, and at parturition. *British Medical Journal*, **1**, 1188

Short, R. V. (1976). The evolution of human reproduction. *Proceedings of the Royal Society of London B*, **195**, 3

Short, R. V. and Baird, D. T. (Eds.) (1976). *Contraceptives of the Future*. (London: The Royal Society)

Short, R. V. and Drife, J. O. (1977). The aetiology of mammary cancer in man and animals. *Symposia of the Zoological Society of London*, **41**, 211

World Health Organization. Special programme of research, development and research training in human reproduction. 6th Annual Report, November 1977

14

Law and planned parenthood

John Paxman
and
Rebecca Cook

INTRODUCTION 228

CONTRACEPTION 228
The prescription requirement 229
Restrictions on the place of sale or distribution 232
Insertion of IUDs 233

VOLUNTARY STERILIZATION 235
Relation of criminal statutes to voluntary sterilization 235
The lack of specific provisions prohibiting voluntary sterilization 237
Trends in laws on voluntary sterilization 238
What makes sterilization voluntary? 240

ABORTION 241
The law on abortion 241
Indications 241
Legal provisions governing the accessibility of abortion services 242
Application, interpretation or change of abortion laws 245

MENSTRUAL REGULATION 250

CONCLUSIONS 252

INTRODUCTION

In a recent provocative article entitled 'The law against family planning', Tunkel sets for himself the task of showing that 'the law as expressed is hostile to the use of modern family planning techniques and the introduction of new ones'. He proves equal to his challenge by demonstrating in a compelling way how the law hinders rather than helps the development and deployment of family planning methods by creating unnecessary ambiguities, contradictions and prohibitions, i.e. 'barriers and bottlenecks'. There is nothing new in this.

That the law creates 'barriers and bottlenecks' to service-orientated family planning programmes has been more than a suspicion since the early years of this century, when pioneers like Marie Stopes began agitating for wider use of family planning methods.

The initial observation that the law 'as expressed' is 'against' family planning is correct, in the sense that the law tends to inhibit rather than promote. Pace-setting innovation is not often thought of as the law's strong suit. The law naturally tends to follow, rather than precede, many of the advances discussed thus far in this book. And the task of changing law is laborious and time-consuming. Where family planning is concerned the law has tagged along behind practice.

But that is only one half of the picture. Tunkel also outlines alternatives which may be developed in relation to the law 'as expressed'. Because the law can exert so much control over how family planning services are provided, the positive role it can take in facilitating family planning is obviously important. Slow as the law is to adapt to fast-moving developments, legal innovations have been made. In many instances the law 'as expressed' has been interpreted in such a way as to make family planning services more widely available. Many laws relating to planned parenthood have been changed in the past decade or alternative legal approaches developed.

The aims of this chapter are, first, to explore the ways in which law restrains service-orientated family planning programmes and, second, to explain how these restraints may be eliminated, overcome or avoided by using law in an imaginative way.

CONTRACEPTION

The need for a doctor's prescription and the restriction of sales to pharmacies are the major legal restrictions placed on the distribution of contraceptives, particularly orals. The rationales supporting the two requirements are closely linked. Argument has it that they are essential for controlling dangerous drugs and poisons which, if used indiscriminately, could otherwise threaten human health. At first glance, the theory behind the approach seems laudable. However, rigid adherence to these requirements, particularly in relation to contraception, has been roundly criticized as inappropriate when the minimal risks of Pill use are weighed against the benefits. Clinically, there is a growing feeling that contraceptives should be made available in simpler ways, as prescription by a doctor and sale by a pharmacist contribute little *per se* to the avoidance of risks related to Pill use. It has been shown (see Chapter 5, for example) that suitably selected and specially trained workers can distribute the Pill safely after obtaining an adequate history from a potential user.

The prescription requirement

One of the traditional statutorily protected functions of a doctor is to prescribe medications for the treatment of human diseases and disorders. Because the Pill and contraceptive injections are normally included in the list of 'potentially harmful drugs' which can be distributed only on prescription, doctors control their flow to the consuming public. In combination, these laws create an effective bottleneck in family planning.

The following generalizations can be made about the prescription requirement. First, it is premised on the availability of doctors to administer it. While in countries where the doctor per capita ratios are relatively high the requirement may not impose an inhibiting effect on the availability of contraceptives, it is in countries where the doctor per capita ratio is low that the requirement acts as the greatest barrier. Stepan and Kellogg observed in their excellent study of laws on contraception that:

'It is surprising how frequently laws relating to the distribution of the Pill fail to reflect, through some degree of flexibility, either the basic factor of the inaccessibility of physicians or urgent demographic pressures. Thus, the law is virtually the same in West Germany and in Nigeria where in a 61 million population, one physician must take care of 40 000 people.'

In many countries it is not unusual to find that the rural populations (which not infrequently reach 80% of the total) live out their lives virtually without any exposure to the care of a doctor. The question is straightforward: Is it reasonable to deny access to contraceptive protection simply because of the prescription requirement? Obviously, viable alternative solutions must be found – solutions which take into account the original purpose of the requirement, the comparatively low risk to health of contraception (including the Pill), the availability of health personnel and the possible consequences of legal change.

Second, the universality of the doctor's prescription requirement is gradually eroding. Over the past 5 years the trend towards changing the prescription requirements for contraceptives has gained considerable momentum. Two basic approaches have been used. Either appropriately trained health and auxiliary personnel have been authorized to prescribe and distribute contraceptives, or the prescription requirement for orals has been eliminated altogether. In summary, the current situation can be described as follows:

No prescription for oral contraceptives required: Antigua, Bangladesh, Grenada, Hong Kong, Iraq, Jamaica, Nepal, Pakistan.

Prescription for oral contraceptives required either by trained health or auxiliary personnel, such as midwives and nurses, or by government authorized personnel, such as field staff workers, when under medical supervision or under a doctor's standing orders: Malaysia, Morocco, Chile, Republic of Korea, South Africa, Sri Lanka, Sweden, the Philippines and Thailand.

Doctor's prescription for oral contraceptives required for the first time only; subsequent resupply provided on a continuing basis by the dispenser on request of the consumer: Fiji, Barbados.

Initial doctor's prescription for 12 months or more, interim supply available from non-doctors: Brazil, Tunisia.

Apropos of the prescription requirement, the IPPF Central Medical Committee observed five years ago that:

'The limitation of oral contraceptive distribution to a doctor's prescription makes the method geographically, economically and sometimes culturally inaccessible to many women. As a consequence, deaths and sickness of women and children, which might otherwise be avoided by the voluntary limitation of fertility, continue . . . The Committee believes that whoever normally meets the health needs of the community, whether doctor, nurse, traditional midwife, pharmacist or storekeeper, can be an appropriate person to distribute oral contraceptives.'

Third, although the prescription requirement still predominates, there is ample evidence that it is widely ignored. In a growing number of countries the requirement is honoured more in the breach, and the *de facto* situation differs considerably from the *de jure*. According to Stepan and Kellogg, this is true in Brazil, Egypt, Ghana, Indonesia, Ivory Coast, Lebanon, Malaysia, Mexico, Panama, the Philippines, Thailand, Turkey and Venezuela. To these may also be added at the very minimum, Bolivia, Colombia, Ecuador, El Salvador, Malaysia and Nigeria. In all of these countries the Pill, as well as other medicaments, are readily available, at least in metropolitan areas, without prescription and little attempt is made by the authorities to stop this. Yet the prescription barrier still inhibits accessibility among the poor and in rural areas. Over-the-counter contraceptives are too expensive for many people to buy, but international agencies will not supply free or subsidized Pills if this is contrary to prescription requirements. For example, in Sri Lanka social marketing of Pills has lagged behind that of condoms because of prescription needs (Chapter 8).

Despite some changes, the doctor prescription requirement remains the greatest barrier to the wider distribution of certain contraceptives. Until this is altered, other ways of working within the technical limits of the prescription requirement must be sought. The following are suggested as approaches which facilitate wider distribution of oral contraceptives and at the same time save valuable doctor time, at least within the traditional clinic setting.

The technique of 'standing orders'

Under this approach the doctor in charge of the clinic issues 'standing orders' to appropriately trained health and auxiliary personnel on how and when to issue the Pill. This is accomplished by giving them a short list of questions they should ask the woman during screening. If the woman answers 'no' to all the questions, the distributor may issue the Pill; if the woman answers 'yes' to any one of the questions, she will be referred to a doctor for further consultation.

The technique of signed prescriptions

At the beginning of the week, the doctor presents the health and auxiliary personnel on the staff with a prescription pad of blank, signed prescriptions along with standing orders or instructions indicating which kind of women can receive oral contraceptives and under what conditions. They are then allowed to prescribe the Pill under the standing orders by using the signed prescription sheets from the pad.

The technique of countersigning prescriptions

Under this system, trained health and auxiliary personnel write the prescription and the doctor countersigns it. This technique is particularly appropriate for programmes with a large number of trained midwives and nurses but few doctors. As with the other techniques, because the trained staff can usually spend more time with the women than the doctor, they get a better response, thus enabling better care.

The technique of long-term prescriptions

The human resources available for the distribution of oral contraceptives may be more wisely spent if long-term prescriptions are used, thereby saving valuable doctor time. This technique involves prescriptions made out for 12 months or more after initial screening by the doctor. Subsequent refills of the prescription are accomplished without the necessity of seeing the doctor again. Once the 12 months have passed, the woman sees the doctor for a check-up and a new prescription.

Restrictions on place of sale or distribution

The restrictions on place of sale and distribution of drugs and devices, found in so many pharmaceutical laws, limit access to contraceptives (e.g. Pills, condoms, foams and jellies) particularly where pharmacies are far away from the consumers. Such requirements cannot help but have a negative impact on contraceptive use. Since potential users in many parts of the world are persons of rather modest means and mobility, they tend to purchase needed commodities (e.g. food or medicine) in frequent, small purchases at shops very near their residences. For this reason, among others, any restrictions which reduce the accessibility of contraceptive outlets make the task of providing continuing contraceptive services much more difficult. Furthermore, the usual restrictions, i.e. sale-in-pharmacy under registered pharmacist's supervision only, have their greatest negative impact in the non-urban areas, where most reliance must or ought to be placed on the use of non-doctor community-based personnel for contraceptive distribution.

Because oral contraceptives are usually subject to prescription, the point of commercial distribution is often restricted to pharmacies. Yet, some countries restrict the commercial distribution of non-prescription contraceptives as well. For example, the 1967 French legislation on contraception required that all sales of contraceptives take place 'exclusively in pharmacies'. This was the rule in France until as recently as 1974.

Various approaches may be taken to reduce the obstacles presented by the sale-in-pharmacy requirement. Special exceptions to the rule could be made which permit other kinds of public or commercial outlets to sell or distribute contraceptives, thereby expanding the network of distribution points. In the public sector, government clinics are usually authorized to distribute on prescription a variety of medicaments, including contraceptives, as part of a government's public health services. This tends to increase the outlets. The key is to use this sort of power to authorize distribution at privately operated clinics and distribution points. In Chile, for example, contraceptives may be distributed at any location authorized by the National Health Services. Authorization could also be extended to health and auxiliary personnel to sell or distribute contraceptives during visits to their clients' homes. This is a variation on what has come to be known as community-based distribution programmes. Its complement is to permit distribution of contraception through normal commercial channels by special distributors in the community setting. Community-based distribution is a recent innovation which holds great promise. In short, the pharmacy sale requirement could be waived for free or subsidized community distribution or government workers; private clinics and certain non-doctor health workers could be authorized to undertake distribution.

However, even where there are many distribution points, the effect on the use of non-doctors in the private sector may be negated by the requirement of doctor authorization or supervision. This fact accentuates the need to orchestrate an increase in the distribution points with an expansion in the types of personnel authorized to handle contraceptives. The Thai example is useful here. In Thailand during 1970–71 only 350 clinics were authorized to distribute oral contraceptives in the National Health Service, because of a regulation which required a physician's prescription prior to issuance. By permitting specially trained auxiliary midwives to distribute the Pill, the number of outlets was increased to nearly 4000. The number of acceptors increased almost four-fold simply because the method became more accessible. The more recent dramatic growth in Pill use at a village level (Chapters 5 and 6) is based on an extension of this same principle.

In the end, the rationale for limiting distribution outlets for any contraceptive is closely linked to the presence or absence of the doctor's prescription requirement. If the need for the prescription requirement can be shown to be inappropriate and the requirement either eliminated or modified, as has happened in many countries, then there is less justification for controlling the number and nature of the distribution outlets. Curiously, however, some of the countries that have eliminated or altered the prescription requirement have kept the one on pharmacy sales, as in Fiji. Such an inconsistency is not only puzzling but somewhat irrational given the circumstances in those countries, particularly in areas where there are no pharmacies.

Insertion of IUDs

The legal requirements concerning the insertion of IUDs differ somewhat from the mere prescription or distribution of the Pill or other contraceptives for the simple reason that IUDs cannot be self-administered. They must be inserted by trained personnel with special skills and knowledge, though that does not mean that it has to be done solely by doctors. As with other forms of contraceptives, the main problem is that there is a shortage of people trained to provide the service. Essentially, three legal approaches have been taken.

1. As a general rule laws and regulations do not specifically regulate IUD insertions. However, the typical pattern has been to assume that an IUD insertion is a medical procedure which, as a matter of traditional medical practice, not law, falls solely upon a doctor. The amendments to the Eugenic Protection Law in Japan, however, codify the notion by stating that 'the act of inserting a contraceptive device in the cavity of the uterus shall not be performed by any person other than a doctor'. (Curiously, the provision existed before the IUD was authorized for use in Japan and may have referred to a diaphragm.) In most countries the situation is merely ambiguous and there is no specific prohibition on IUD insertions by non-doctors. Many countries do not frown on non-doctor insertions, as long as those who do it are properly trained.

2. There is a growing trend, principally in parts of the world where there are shortages of doctors, though not restricted to them, toward authorizing non-doctor personnel to perform IUD insertions. All indications are that non-doctors can be trained to insert IUDs safely and efficiently. The South Korean Maternal and Child Health Law, No. 2514 of 8 February 1973 states in Section 7 that the 'insertion of intra-uterine contraceptives shall be performed only by a physician or those who are designated by presidential decree'. The Presidential Ordinance No. 6713 of 28 May 1973 indicates that the category of designated persons includes: '. . . licensed midwives or nurses who have been trained in such courses as prescribed by the Minister of Health and Social Affairs for more than two months . . .'. Of course, midwives in Pakistan have been used to insert IUDs for nearly a decade. And IUDs were 'the first contraceptive method introduced in China on a large scale'. Most of the insertions there are done by trained nurses, midwives or 'barefoot doctors'. In addition, Chile, Sweden and the Philippines have authorized properly trained non-physician personnel to insert OUDs, and it is a practice in Britain and certain States of the USA.

3. France is one of the few countries with a detailed law on the subject of IUD insertion. Among the provisions of the 1967 law was the following: 'Intra-uterine contraceptives may be inserted *by a physician* only in a hospital establishment, an approved treatment centre, or in conformity with conditions to be determined by public administrative regulations.'

Initially then, IUD insertions were restricted to public or private hospitals with either gynaecological or maternity departments or a genetic counselling service. Under more recent regulations, physicians were given authority to perform insertions outside the hospital setting, in clinics or surgeries, if they received approval to do so from the local medical inspector. The recently revised Hungarian regulations insist that only trained gynaecologists insert IUDs. Where such specifically rigid requirements exist it is difficult to see a role for non-doctors in insertions.

Part of the problem of utilizing non-doctors for IUD insertions is that it will be argued that they are encroaching on the practice of medicine. Moreover, nursing and midwifery legislation may also preclude activity of this type. There is little reason to adhere rigidly to this view. For one thing, doctors are legally entitled to delegate tasks to non-doctor personnel. This approach can be used to advantage in a majority of countries. Delegation requires that the doctor properly train and supervise the personnel he is to utilize. That should not be too much of a burden as any system which uses non-doctors should make provision for supervision and referrals. In the end, it is the restrictive attitude of doctors themselves, as much as the law, which inhibits efforts to provide IUD insertion services.

VOLUNTARY STERILIZATION

Voluntary sterilization for family planning purposes is becoming an increasingly popular method. Recent studies assert that it is the single most used method of contraception. Even so, the law has sadly lagged behind in addressing the issues. Since voluntary sterilization for purely contraceptive purposes is a relatively new phenomenon, many countries do not have laws which specifically regulate the procedure. In the large number of countries without any statutory law specifically against voluntary sterilization the operation is probably legal, even though it may not be common medical practice. The greatest area of present confusion involves attempts to ascertain whether the criminal law applies a bar to voluntary sterilization for family planning purposes.

Relation of criminal statutes to voluntary sterilization

Most criminal statutes neither *specifically* prohibit nor permit voluntary sterilization. Hence, there is some uncertainty as to whether the law applies. The apprehension on the part of family planners is that the law prohibits the procedure, and rather than risk possible criminal penalties they abstain from offering sterilization services. Indeed, the predominant legal view in some countries considers sterilization a form of intentional infliction of grievous bodily harm, assault, or mayhem, as expressed in Common Law systems, or of *'coups et blessures volontaires'* (intentional wounds and injuries), as expressed in Civil Law codes. Such views have a chilling impact on attempts to offer sterilization services.

Many countries, however, are now moving to resolve these uncertainties by removing doubts as to what the law says about this subject. Article 262 of the Revised Penal Code of the Philippines imposes penalties 'upon any person who shall intentionally mutilate another by depriving him, either totally or partially, of some organ essential for reproduction'. In an opinion dated 17 September 1973, Secretary of Justice Vicente Abad Santos answered the question whether the statute prohibits voluntary sterilization. Since, he observed, methods of sterilization (tubal ligation and vasectomy) 'do not involve lopping or clipping off the organs of reproduction of both sexes', as may be the case with castration, but 'are effected by the closing of a pair of small tubes in either the man or the woman so that the sperm and ovum cannot meet', they should not be regarded as 'mutilation within the contemplation of Article 262'. Similar interpretations have been developed in other countries. In Singapore the Voluntary Sterilization Act, 1974 contains a provision which states, to avoid doubt, that 'sexual sterilization by a registered medical practitioner shall not constitute a 'grievous hurt' within the meaning of the Penal Code'.

Voluntariness is another important dimension of the problem and offers another way of overcoming the legal barriers to voluntary sterilization. In many countries, if the 'victim' consents, the person inflicting the so-called 'injury' cannot be held criminally responsible. This is an important exception to the usual rule. It leaves room for surgical procedures to be performed without fear of penal sanctions. For example, Article 24 of the Penal Code of South Korea provides:

'Conduct which infringes a legal interest shall not be punishable, except as otherwise provided by law, where the consent of someone who is authorized to dispose of such an interest is obtained.'

Similar provisions are found in the penal codes of Ethiopia and Greece, as well as those of India, Pakistan, Sri Lanka, Burma, Malaysia and Uruguay, to name but a few.

On the other hand, in France, Belgium and some other Civil Law countries, the consent of the 'victim' to 'grave bodily injury' does not free the surgeon performing sterilization operation from criminal liability. In the celebrated '*Bordeaux sterilisateurs*' case of 1937, a group of French people were accused of advocating and practising voluntary sterilization on ideological grounds.

Although the accused were not authorized physicians, and could have been prosecuted on other grounds, the decision was based on the principle that the consent of those individuals was irrelevant to the criminal responsibility of the accused, on the theory that the patients 'could not authorize anyone to violate, on their persons, the rules governing the public order'. This attitude prevails into the present; in theory it poses a rather formidable obstacle.

The degree of confusion which exists in many countries is indicated by the fact that the laws ostensibly applicable are the criminal laws on assault and severe bodily injury which equate the work of a skilled physician on a willing patient under clinical conditions with a brutal assault. A more reasonable approach is taken in some African countries with an English Common Law background (Ghana, Nigeria, Tanzania and Zambia). There voluntary sterilization is simply considered a 'surgical operation', which, if done in good faith for the intended benefit of the patient, is not the subject of criminal liability. This is a sensible way to resolve the question of criminal liability and at the same time avoid the present confusion in many countries.

The lack of specific provisions prohibiting voluntary sterilization

The lack of *specific* provisions in criminal codes concerning the legality or illegality of voluntary sterilization calls to mind the doctrine, *nullum crimen, nulla pœna sine lege.* Loosely translated, it means that an act is considered criminal only when it is stated to be so in a criminal code. This precept of criminal law, common to virtually all legal systems of the world, can be applied with advantage to voluntary sterilization. Accordingly, voluntary sterilization would be legal in those countries whose laws do not expressly forbid it.

This approach would not work where laws prohibit voluntary sterilization under any circumstances, as in Italy. Section 552 of the Penal Code of 19 October 1930 provides:

'Whoever performs acts on persons of either sex, with their consent, intended to render them incapable of procreating, will be punished by imprisonment from six months to two years and with a fine from eight to forty thousand lira. Whoever gives consent to those acts being performed on himself shall suffer the same punishment.'

It should be noted, not to overstate the case, that where voluntary sterilization is prohibited, either *per se* or by analogy to the infliction of 'grievous bodily harm', the actual prosecution or conviction of the doctors or patients is rare (the last known case in France occurred in 1937, and that in Austria in 1934) or unknown (Chile, Indonesia, Costa Rica, and Colombia). That is not to say that sterilization for family planning purposes is legal because no prosecutions have taken place. It only emphasizes the disparity between what the law says and what may go on in practice. As long as restrictive laws are on the books, the threat of punishment must be seen as an inhibiting factor, however.

Trends in laws on voluntary sterilization

On the whole, there is a general trend towards liberalizing laws on voluntary sterilization. Where laws specifically authorize voluntary sterilization, they generally prescribe certain pre-conditions to the performance of the operation. The following are examples of what may be encountered; any or all may create barriers, some more severe than others, yet at the same time they may afford special protections to those who require the service.

Waiting period

Some laws require a waiting period between the request for a voluntary sterilization operation and the actual operation. This provides an opportunity to reconsider the decision and may be seen as an attempt to eliminate possible coercion. This feature of the law has generated much discussion in the United States of late, where regulations governing federally-funded voluntary sterilization programmes insist on a 30 day waiting period. On the one hand, the principle concerned seems to have been to protect 'welfare mothers' from the coercive practice of insisting that they be sterilized as part of the price for performing an abortion and/or the receipt of welfare benefits. On the other, one can argue that such a requirement leads to a waste of resources and makes getting a sterilization more difficult where no coercion is being applied.

Some countries have set about shortening the waiting period. A 1972 amendment of the Singapore Voluntary Sterilization Act of 1969 reduced the waiting period from thirty to seven days. In the 1974 Act the requirement was eliminated altogether. Conversely, Denmark requires that the operation be performed not later than six months after the authorization so as to ensure speedy delivery of the service or to avoid possible changes of circumstances.

Minimum age

The imposition of a minimum age requirement on applicants for voluntary sterilization is ostensibly designed to protect them from reaching a rash decision with irreversible consequences, only to regret it later in life. The requirement affects the ability to consent. The minimum age is 18 in Denmark (with careful screening of applicants under 21 years of age) and 25 in West Germany (with exceptions for special circumstances, such as if a woman already has four children). In Singapore, the age requirement has been eliminated for some individuals, but is 21 if the person is not married. But in some countries, the age is higher. Depending on national circumstances such a requirement may make sterilization an unattainable choice where marriage has taken place at an early age and desired family size is reached before majority.

Spousal consent

Since the number of children is arguably a matter of concern to both spouses, many laws require that prior to voluntary sterilization, evidence must be submitted showing the spouse's consent to the operation. Such laws exist in Denmark, Japan and many Moslem countries. Japan also requires a form of spousal consent whenever the person, though 'not legally married, possesses marital status' with the applicant. There is growing unease over this requirement on the theory that the woman has the sole right to make decisions relating to her fertility. The RPPF Medical Committee Law Panel have suggested that spousal consent requirements be eliminated as a matter of law.

Facilities

Several laws specifically require that voluntary sterilization operations be performed in hospitals managed or supervised by the government. Examples are Czechoslovakia, Denmark and Singapore. While such requirements appear to be reasonable health measures, as technology becomes simpler they may tend to restrict access to voluntary sterilization.

Minimum number of living children

Some laws require that before an applicant can be given authorization for voluntary sterilization, evidence must be shown that he or she has already a certain number of living children – 5 for Panama, 4 (or 3 if the woman concerned is over 35 years of age) for Czechoslovakia, and 3 for India. In short, proof of fertility is the price one must pay for curtailing fertility by sterilization.

Authorization by an official board

Several countries require the establishment of an official board to receive, review and decide on applications for voluntary sterilization, in all or selected (e.g. if the applicant is under age) cases. There is no unanimity, however, with respect to the size or professional composition of the board, as well as the method for reaching a decision (by majority or unanimity rules). Some countries' experiences indicate that these administrative arrangements make access to services more difficult. Moreover, it has often been said that such decisions should be left to the doctor and patient. To a certain extent these administrative screening procedures are vestiges of the older sterilization laws which dealt with sterilization for therapeutic and eugenic reasons.

What makes sterilization voluntary?

The sterilization we have been discussing is *voluntary* sterilization. The recent furore in India over attempts to enforce a policy favouring compulsory sterilization for certain couples has prodded the world community into looking more closely at the voluntariness of the sterilization services. The fact that the method, at present, is considered irreversible has heightened concern that it be made available in the absence of unnecessary pressure and that recipients are fully informed of the consequences.

In legal terms, the initial responsibility of those who provide voluntary sterilization services is to ensure that the individual gives mature, informed, unpressured consent to the operation, is legally adult, and legally and socially competent to give that consent. If any of these elements are lacking, the sterilization is not voluntary. Consent is nothing more than an informed choice. To this end, those providing sterilization have a legal responsibility to ensure that the individual seeking the operation receives, in a way that is appropriate to the cultural conditions, and understands, information about the procedure. Such information should include a discussion of the availability of alternative temporary methods of family planning, the advisability of the procedure as a contraceptive method, a description of the techniques used in the procedure itself and its long and short-term benefits and risks to health. It should be made clear to the individual that at present sterilization should be considered an irreversible procedure. However, it should be stressed that the operation does not necessarily guarantee the prevention of pregnancy in every case, particularly during the immediate post-sterilization stage for males. In the case of male sterilization, the individual should be notified of the need to use other preventative measures in the immediate post-sterilization phase, and if possible, be provided with the means to do so, such as condoms. As an additional protection, patients should be told that they are free to change their minds about being sterilized, and that if they do so no benefits will be withdrawn from them.

ABORTION

The law on abortion

Current abortion laws take a variety of forms, impose a variety of restrictions and differ considerably in their content. Nevertheless, certain general provisions and legislative patterns emerge. It appears, for instance, that abortion laws affect:

* (a) a person who attempts to procure and/or procures an abortion, whether that person is medically qualified or not;
* (b) a woman who attempts to procure and/or procures her own abortion, acting alone or with another person, in (a) above;
* (c) a person who furnishes the means to procure abortion, to someone in (a) and/or (b) above.
* (d) persons who refer women to an abortion facility, physician or abortionist.

Laws differ in the degrees and extents to which they permit women to choose abortion. Most laws, however, are similar in seeking protection of women's health against unqualified interference, whether by surgical intervention, manipulation, or administration of toxic substances. Different legal sytems respond differently to reasons for seeking abortion. Many reflect ambivalence, opposing abortion in principle but having sympathy for known women who find specific pregnancies unendurable. Ambivalence clouds both the definition of the legitimate grounds for abortion and the indications on which legitimate abortion services may be provided.

Indications

It goes without saying that there is no uniformity among abortion laws. Different countries have selected the justifications for legal termination of pregnancy from within the following range of indications:

* risk to the life of the woman;
* risk to the woman's health (both physical and mental health) from continuation of pregnancy, meaning risk beyond that normally associated with pregnancy (the therapeutic indication);

* some degree of likely physical or mental impairment of a child if born (the fetal indication);
* pregnancy by rape or incest (the judicial indication);
* the effect of childbirth upon the health and welfare of the woman and her existing children and family (the social, socio-medical or socio-economic indication);
* jeopardy to the social position of the woman or her family (the family indication);
* failure of a routinely employed contraceptive means (the contraceptive indication);
* on request (usually during the first trimester).

Legal provisions governing the accessibility of abortion services

Over the past 10 years there has been a noticeable trend towards extending the indications upon which abortions can be made available. As a first step, this trend is encouraging, but there is evidence that many of the changes sought in the law have not been brought about for fault of implementation. The services made legal in theory have not been made available in practice. Legitimizing termination of pregnancy does not in itself compel administrative authorities controlling health resources to meet the existing demand for abortion, nor does it ensure availability of services at the earliest possible stage of pregnancy. Additionally, requirements within the law itself may make the services virtually inaccessible.

Beyond indications, the law affects the availability of abortion services in that it determines:

* who should perform abortions (e.g. doctors, nurses, trained health and auxiliary personnel);
* where abortions should be performed (e.g. approved hospitals or clinics, on an inpatient or outpatient basis);
* what approval procedures should be followed (e.g. medical concurrence, such as by a second opinion or an abortion committee or parental or spousal consent); and
* what conscience clauses can be invoked.

Such provisions may be responsible in part for limiting the impact of so-called liberal laws.

Who should perform abortions?

The usual prescription is to insist that abortions be performed only by registered medical practitioners. Some laws require that only specialists perform abortions. A number of contending arguments emerge from legislation which confines procedures to medical practitioners and from that which requires special qualifications of practitioners. It may seem difficult to oppose concentrating abortion procedures exclusively in the hands of qualified physicians. Protection of the health of women is an interest of the highest individual and social priority.

The argument in favour of ensuring high standards seems compelling, especially since adverse reactions to routine procedures may in principle arise in any individual case. Nevertheless, the argument can be overstated, and its emphasis upon excellence has been found both to condemn the safe and good and sometimes to disregard the governing realities. If all medical procedures required performance by only the most highly skilled, many fewer could be undertaken than in fact are, and the requisite skills would be more difficult to develop. Childbirth itself, which in countries with liberal abortion laws presents a greater hazard to female health than early pregnancy termination, is not generally surrounded by special legal requirements relating to the qualification of physicians. Moreover, leading physicians delegate many procedures, for which they remain medically responsible, to their staffs. They advise, supervise, and are at hand, of course, in the event of emergency, but do not attend in person. The simplicity and safety of early abortion and menstrual regulation are noted in Chapter 11 and contrasted with those of illegal operation.

In both developed and developing regions of the world properly trained midwives, public health nurses and comparable health and auxiliary personnel perform many medical procedures and can also conduct abortion procedures early in pregnancy under adequate supervision. An advantage of their involvement may be their ability to provide an equal or a higher quality of pre- and post-abortion care and counselling than a busy physician can offer, thereby securing better and perhaps more confidential overall patient management. They already play an important role in fertility control, including menstrual regulation to which the earliest abortion is analogous. Further, as research produces non-surgical abortifacients with controllable side-effects, and as physicians' proximity to their employment can therefore be reduced, effective management can be projected along more extended lines of delegation.

Legally restricting medical services to the most scarce and costly personnel may prejudice service to the community. It may be appropriate in some countries to use *standing orders* in hospitals, clinics, and primary health centres to achieve appropriate delegations of functions to trained health and auxiliary personnel. The alternative is to make such procedures unavailable to those who have no access to a doctor or who are unable to pay the cost involved.

Where should abortions be performed?

Laws either restrict the provision of abortion services to specified institutions or leave such directions to the discretion of the health profession. Differences between standards required of facilities undertaking outpatient and inpatient services are becoming important as technology advances and barriers to early abortion are removed. The argument that has favoured detailed legal supervision of the site of abortion services is that it promotes a high quality of care and reduces or accommodates emergencies. The argument on the other side is that regulations can exaggerate administrative and penal concerns irrationally. Early abortion is safer than normal childbirth. There is every reason to believe that menstrual regulation can be carried out safely in a doctor's surgery. But regulations have tended to ignore these developments.

What approval procedures should be followed?

Second doctor's opinion, board approval, etc. – Approval procedures vary from requiring the approval of the requesting woman and the practising professional (e.g. in Tunisia), to requiring additional doctors' opinions (e.g. in UK) or the approval of a board (e.g. in Canada). Some jurisdictions such as in India and East Germany require special approval only after a specified time period, usually the first trimester of pregnancy.

The purpose behind abortion legislation requiring an approval procedure is to authenticate that the abortion is performed only on the basis of a legal indication. The fact that the particular indication approved usually does not have to be agreed on by the two or more professionals, suggests that the procedure is in fact neither aimed at improving health care nor for the purpose of providing pre-abortion and post-abortion counselling. The approval, more often than not, serves to insulate those who make the decision.

Where specific approval requirements exist, they increase delay and work against the availability of services at the earliest possible stage of pregnancy. Experience shows that legal requirements for approval procedures result in unequal applications of the law, particularly against poor women and women in rural areas. The legal requirement of another opinion is different, of course, from a medical decision in a particular case to consulting another physician for his clinical opinion.

Consent requirements – Few abortion laws mention consent, although one or two state in terms what is evident without expression, that the woman involved must consent to performance of the procedure upon her. The abortion laws that do mention consent require either parental or spousal consent.

Evidence shows that where the consent of anyone other than the woman alone is required, it often leads to delay, with an attendant rise in the risks of the procedure. It also places a woman's future health at another's disposal. Even so, where it is beneficial for family harmony to encourage the partner's and/or parent's involvement, it is desirable to allow this, as a matter of practice with the woman's prior consent, but not as a requirement of law.

Conscientious objection clause

Abortion laws often do not adequately deal with those who have conscientious objections to abortion.

Those with religious or other conscientious objections to abortion *per se*, as opposed to objections based on the features of an individual case, should be exempted from participation. This applies equally to doctors, health and auxiliary personnel and those who would normally be called upon to provide abortion services. The exemption should apply to performance of the procedure itself. It should not justify refusal of auxiliary services, such as post-operative care. In emergency situations, moreover, such clauses have to be waived.

In Yugoslavia, the conscience clause in the law was used to refuse services and was therefore subsequently omitted in the revised law. In order to avoid such abuses and to ensure that those with genuine religious and conscientious objections do not have to participate in the provision of abortion services, those with such objections have the ethical responsibility to refer women to others who will provide the care; they cannot simply abandon the patient.

Application, interpretation or change of abortion laws

Application of the law

Abortion law may be the most stoutly defended and least enforced law on national statute books. Its symbolic role in defence of the defenceless and as tribute to human life at its inception affords it a powerful emotive appeal. Instances of enforcement, however, are notoriously unsuccessful.

Nonetheless, in many jurisdictions, conscientious doctors are hesitant to proceed in providing abortion, or even abortion related services, because of fear of prosecution. Such fears are invariably unfounded, as often those responsible for initiating public prosecutions will only move to prosecute unqualified practitioners or obviously exploitive physicians. In countries where the law is unclear, public prosecutors use their discretion to choose the cases where there is clear evidence of negligence or unqualified practice.

Discretion is the key to application. In certain legal systems, particularly those based on Civil Law, the prosecutor has a right to use his discretion, deciding to prosecute or not under the principle of opportunity. The appropriate legal authority, for instance the public prosecutor or the Attorney General, has the power to declare that prosecution is not to be brought under his authority against a registered medical practitioner, performing medical termination of pregnancy in what he regards, in good faith, as the best interests of his patient.

Such an approach would go a long way towards clarifying the legal status of abortion and at the same time protect the providers of legitimate abortion services. A variation of this approach was used in France prior to the abortion law reform in 1975. There M. Giscard d'Estaing announced that women who sought abortions would no longer be prosecuted under the draconian 1920 statute in force at the time. That decision served as a prelude to change.

Methods of protecting and reassuring providers of abortion services

Good faith checklist – Prosecutions will probably not be brought against providers of abortion services if they can show that such services have been provided in good faith and with the best interests of the woman in mind. In some jurisdictions, particularly Common Law jurisdictions, a physician who acts in good faith does not commit and cannot be convicted of an illegal abortion. Good faith is established by evidence which details the conscientious examination of the applicant to establish a medical basis for the legal indications.

Despite the uniqueness of each case, a uniform checklist could be developed by the Ministry of Health or, if drafted by other means, be approved by them as a guideline. Such a checklist should identify the points a physician should cover in questioning and examining a woman (areas of physical health, mental health, existing children's health, socio-economic conditions, congenital problems, etc., depending on the scope of the law). If a completed checklist, containing suitable detail, were to be carefully prepared for each procedure, the doctor's good faith could be legally evidenced, and his susceptibility to prosecution reduced.

Referral letters and case histories – Keeping referral letters and related data, like case histories, is another way to 'protect' the doctor. If a full case history exists and is available, it is most likely that legitimate health reasons for a procedure will be contained in that history. This will also confirm some professional consensus on the medical suitability of abortion in the patient's circumstances.

Clarification of the law – Confusion often exists about what an abortion law really says. One way to avoid this is to ask law officers to clarify the details of existing law. Even where no checklist is developed, they can be asked whether present law permits abortion where life or health are at risk, what degree of danger to health justifies the procedure, whether rape or incest are permissible grounds and whether, for instance, a girl's young age (such as 14) justifies abortion. Such a step proved useful, for example, in Western Australia. There are drawbacks, of course, to asking the authorities, particularly if their interpretation of the law is narrow, but it may provide an opportunity to take an innovative view of how the law is to be applied in practice.

Low fees – Low fees, consistent with the means of the woman, are also evidence of good faith. While it is difficult to set a price, in relative terms, it has been suggested that abortion should not cost more than a week's disposable income of the woman. An exorbitant or exploitive fee suggests that it contains an inducement to take the risk of acting illegally.

Failure to provide service – When indications exist upon which medical opinion would consider abortion necessary or justified, for instance as shown in the evolving medical literature, physicians and health facilities are obliged to consider abortion as a legitimate medical option. Practitioners and facilities may not have the option of *not* performing, or of not considering performing, an abortion. Many doctors and facilities decline involvement in abortion for purely self-protective purposes; they do not want to risk involvement with the law. But in adopting this attitude, they do not necessarily avoid liability. In rejecting a medical option on non-medical grounds, they may be sued for negligence and if the pregnant woman's health is damaged through continued pregnancy and/or giving birth, they may be liable for criminal negligence. If death follows a non-medical refusal of abortion, liability for manslaughter by criminal negligence may arise. Legally, therefore, the medical option of *not* considering abortion an alternative in reality never arises, unless (as is rarely the case) the law absolutely prohibits abortion in any and every case.

Legality of treatment of incomplete abortion – Doctors hesitate to proceed with the treatment of incomplete abortion and women fail to seek proper treatment of incomplete abortion because they think it is illegal, particularly where the law is restrictive. This attitude prevails principally because of the fear of detection and prosecution. The treatment of incomplete abortion is legal. The treatment of incomplete abortion in most countries is governed by the law relating to medical procedures and, in general, does not usually fall under the rules stated in the abortion law. All that would normally be required is the consent of the woman being treated. Ethical issues aside, failure to treat a woman for an incomplete abortion involves some of the same legal issues discussed in the preceding paragraph.

Equipment – The purchase of equipment by physicians which can be used for abortion as well as for other procedures should not be considered evidence of an intent to commit abortion. Supplying the means to procure abortion may be an offence in the context of a particular illegal abortion, but simply supplying or acquiring a medical (or non-medical) instrument capable of achieving abortion illegally is not evidence that it was supplied or acquired for that purpose. Where such means can have an innocent employment, in this case use for other obstetric or gynaecological procedures, the general presumption of the accused's innocence prevails, and no adverse inference can be drawn from the mere fact of the physician's possession, or indeed use, of such equipment.

Options for legal interpretation or reform

A number of options, in addition to those discussed above, are available to those who wish to expand the availability of abortion services. These include the following:

Definition of health – In many countries a statute which directly relates to the health of the woman is interpreted in the light of the purpose of protecting the health. For example, although a statute may permit abortion to 'preserve the life of the woman' this can often be interpreted to mean to protect her mental and physical health. The fact that the adverse impact upon her life may not take place immediately does not make it any the less a threat to her life. In effect, 'life' may mean not just physical existence but can encompass the quality of life, which would be adversely affected by continuation of pregnancy.

To avoid problems over the definition of the word 'health', the World Health Organization definition of health might be usefully related to abortion laws:

'Health is a state of complete physical, mental and social well-being and not merely the absence of disease or infirmity.'

By applying such a definition broadly, what are thought to be narrow grounds for abortion can be greatly expanded. But, to be realistic, the WHO definition seems to be a working administrative definition and in that light may not contribute much to the legal debate.

Fundamental principles of possible application – A number of fundamental legal principles exist which may be helpful in applying, interpreting or changing legislative, judicial and administrative provisions relating to abortion law.

* *The right of privacy and integrity.* Applied to abortion, this principle means that the abortion decision is a private matter between the woman and her physician. As such, decisions to undergo an abortion need not be reported to the authorities. There is some tension here between the right of privacy and the criminal law. But where the decision is taken in good faith, the right of privacy should prevail.
* *The principle of necessity.* Criminal liability will not attach to individuals who perform abortions to save 'the life or health of others against imminent danger'. Most systems of criminal law embrace this principle, and many of the leading prosecutions of physicians have been successfully thwarted through the use of this defence.
* *Equal application of laws.* The disparity in the application of abortion laws among different socio-economic groups is easily observed. The ease with which wealthy women can evade the prohibition of abortion, by procuring medical or psychiatric opinions of its necessity or by procuring abortions abroad, leaves only the poor and disadvantageous bound, in fact, by prohibitive law. Laws which distribute the burden unevenly can be attacked.
* *Health care decision-making.* The basic obligation of the physician is to decide, in his clinical judgement, what is best for the health of the patient, and to decide on health grounds only. Where health considerations form the basis of the judgement, the physician can proceed with treatment. From another point of view, decisions not to treat which are based on non-health grounds are improper. To be even-handed, in some cases so too are decisions to treat on non-health grounds.

Test cases – In a number of instances, the above-mentioned principles have played a large part in cases which have tested the abortion law. Test cases have helped to focus on deficiencies in abortion laws and have served to clarify the law favourably (e.g. Bourne (UK), Edgal (Nigeria), Woolnough (New Zealand), Morgentaler (Canada)).

Test cases may take a variety of forms. They may consist of provoking law-enforcement authorities into prosecuting for illegal abortion a physician who has terminated a woman's pregnancy under circumstances he considered medically sound. In this way the limits of the law may become clearer. This is the usual pattern. The danger with it, however, is that it exposes not only the physician, but also the patient, who herself may have committed an offence, to the strains of criminal litigation.

More dramatically, the criminal prohibition of abortion may be attacked as being unconstitutional. This may be done either on the theory that the law violates individual rights, or on the grounds that the law is too vague, e.g. in not separating first trimester abortions from others, or in not separating contraception (where lawful) from abortion.

Extend indications for abortion – One of the obvious ways to achieve wider availability of abortion services is to reform the law outright. This can take two forms:

* Include among the indications for abortion such grounds as health of the woman as defined by WHO, and for additional reasons such as the likelihood of a seriously defective fetus, rape or incest, contraceptive failure, lack of availability of contraceptive services, prevention of unwed motherhood, the protection of the honour of the family, and/or the socio-economic and socio-medical effect of another child in the family.
* Allow abortion on request during the first trimester of pregnancy and for specified indications thereafter.

Decriminalize abortion – The final major option is to decriminalize abortion, that is take it out of the criminal code and make it subject to health care regulations.

* Decriminalize procedures done very early in pregnancy when abortion is most safely done and is ethically and emotionally most acceptable.
* Repeal anti-abortion laws, to permit regulation of abortion according to the existing practice applied to other surgical procedures.

MENSTRUAL REGULATION

As the technology for fertility regulation has become increasingly advanced, laws have not kept pace. There is no better way to emphasize this fact than to look at the case of menstrual regulation. The recent development of the menstrual regulation techniques is having an impact on fertility regulation (Chapter 11). Basically, there are two means for performing menstrual regulation: (1) use of prostaglandins – substances which are naturally present at menstruation and childbirth – and (2) the use of a flexible polyethylene cannula aspirator. Aside from the simplicity and safety of the method, the value of this procedure is that it can be used to ensure a non-pregnant state prior to the medical determination of pregnancy. Many proponents of the menstrual regulation procedure are urging that it be used during the 2 weeks immediately following a missed period. Thus, a woman who suspects that she is pregnant can ask to have the procedure performed and afterwards be guaranteed that she is not, because any embryo which may have begun formation will have been eliminated.

The use of the technique raises several legal issues. How the law affects menstrual regulation depends on how the law defines abortion. While menstrual regulation certainly can be used as a *licit* method of pregnancy termination within the framework of liberalized laws, there are two sub-categories of laws which particularly relate to menstrual regulation: those which (a) make abortion, or the attempt, a crime whether or not the woman is pregnant, and those which (b) expressly or implicitly require proof of pregnancy as an element of criminal offence.

Those laws which make abortion, or its attempt, a crime where the intent for intervening is to provoke a miscarriage, whether or not the woman is pregnant, are derived from two models. One is the restrictive legislation passed in England in 1861; the other is found within the French Penal Code. Despite the fact that both countries have since liberalized their own abortion statutes, the influence of these nineteenth century laws is still in evidence in some Commonwealth countries and in former French colonies. Under these laws, if menstrual regulation is performed with the 'intent' of interrupting a pregnancy, the abortion law is technically violated. If menstrual regulation is used for either therapeutic or diagnostic reasons, it is not. This distinction is useful to family planners.

In other legal systems, particularly those which apply throughout Latin America, actual proof of pregnancy is a prerequisite for a successful abortion prosecution. Without proof of pregnancy, it is said that in the legal sense there can be no abortion, and therefore the law cannot be violated. For this reason, it is possible to defend the performance of menstrual regulation as a legal procedure for women who seek help soon after missing a period but before pregnancy can be verified clinically.

It must be emphasized that there have been no test cases in any part of the world relating to the legal status of menstrual regulation *per se*. In the absence of any precedent, doctors and others will have to depend on legal advice they may be given concerning the application of the abortion law to menstrual regulation. However, the trend seems to be to treat menstrual regulation for the purposes of terminating pregnancy, as falling within the provisions of already existing abortion laws and regulations. Yet there is still some doubt whether these should apply or not. Undoubtedly, further evolution and definition of the legal status of the new option of menstrual regulation in family planning will take place in the future. For the present, it is safe to say the menstrual regulation may be performed legally in many countries in the world, particularly in those which require proof of pregnancy before a prosecution for abortion can go forward.

CONCLUSIONS

Although the law has often been used in a negative way in relation to human fertility regulation, it can be utilized in such a way as to resolve rather than create problems. There is much to be done in this regard. On a global scale the innovative inroads have been slight. To come full circle, Tunkel candidly reminds us that:

'The picture that emerges may seem at times unrealistic, in that family planning activities are seldom interfered with in fact by those who administer the law. Nevertheless, it is important to see the law as the potential hindrance that it is, especially in relation to the new family planning techniques now being developed.'

We must necessarily begin and end with the premise that the law creates 'barriers and bottlenecks'. We cannot ignore what experience has taught us. It is, however, unnecessary to wallow forever in this sort of pessimism. Given the subject matter and the interests to be protected, it is equally unrealistic to expect the law to tolerate a *laissez faire* situation with regard to family planning services. The challenge is to shape the control which the law exerts so as to facilitate rather than hinder family planning programmes.

Bibliography

Cook, R. J. and Dickens, B. M. (1977). A survey of abortion law in Commonwealth countries. In *Three Studies of Abortion Laws in the Commonwealth.* (London: Commonwealth Secretariat)

Cook, R. J. and Dickens, B.M. (1978). A decade of change in abortion law: 1967–77. *American Journal of Public Health,* **68,** 637

Cook, R. J. and Senanayake, P. (eds.) (1978). *The Human Problem of Abortion: The Medico-Legal Dimensions*. The Report of the Ad Hoc Expert Panel on Abortion (London: International Planned Parenthood Federation)

Cook, R. J. (1976). Distribution of oral contraceptives: legal changes and new concepts of preventive care. *American Journal of Public Health,* **66,** 590

International Planned Parenthood Federation (1977). *Family Planning Handbook for Midwives and Nurses*. Second Edition, (London)

International Planned Parenthood Federation (1978). *Family Planning Handbook for Doctors*. Second Edition (London)

International Planned Parenthood Federation (1977). Report of the IPPF Law Panel and the Central Medical Committee on Voluntary Sterilization (in press)

Lee, L. T. and Paxman, J. M. (1975). *Pregnancy and Abortion in Adolescence: Legal Aspects*. Law and Population Monograph Series No. 26, Law and Population Programme, Medford, Massachusetts. Reprinted from *Colum. Human Rights Law Rev.,* **6,** 307

Lee, L. T. and Paxman, J. M. (1975). Legal aspects of the menstrual regulation: some preliminary observations. *Journal of Family Law,* **14,** 181

Paxman, J. M., Lee, L. T. and Hopkins, S. B. (1976). *Expanded Roles for Non-physicians in Fertility Regulation: Legal Perspectives*. Law and Population Monograph Series No. 41, Law and Population Programme, Medford, Massachusetts

Stepan, J. and Kellogg, E. H. (1974). *The World's Laws on Contraceptives,* Law and Population Monograph Series No. 17, Law and Population Programme, Medford, Massachusetts, Reprinted in *American Journal of Comparative Law,* **22,** 615

Stepan, J. and Kellogg, E. H. (1973). *The World's Laws Concerning Voluntary Sterilization for Family Planning Purposes*. Law and Population Monograph Series No. 8, Law and Population Programme, Medford, Massachusetts. Reprinted in *Cal. West. International Law Journal* (1974), **5,** 72

Tunkel, V. (1977). The law against family planning: a Commonwealth survey. In *Three Studies of Abortion Laws in the Commonwealth* (London: Commonwealth Secretariat)

United Nations Fund for Population Activities (1976). *Survey of Contraceptive Laws*. (New York)

World Health Organization (1970–78). *International Digest of Health Legislation* (Geneva)

15

Resources for research

Roy Greep

INTRODUCTION	255
FUNDING	256
Historical perspective	256
The decade of growth and regression	257
Funding outlook and projected needs	261
PROFESSIONAL PERSONNEL AND FACILITIES	263
THE ADVANTAGES AND DISADVANTAGES OF CONDUCTING RESEARCH IN THE DEVELOPING *VIS-À-VIS* THE DEVELOPED NATIONS	263
CONCLUSIONS	264

INTRODUCTION

The resources for research in the reproductive sciences and conception control are at this particular point in time facing an uncertain future. That is an especially enigmatic situation for the reason that research in this area is generally acknowledged to be critical to the solution of some of the most urgent health, social and economic problems facing nations and individuals today. Scientific investigation in this politically sensitive area was long handicapped and delayed by existing taboos of social, cultural and religious nature and became the recipient of expansionary funding only a few years ago. Now that is already declining. Concern over these and other matters relating to the control of human fertility and containment of the expanding population led the Ford Foundation to sponsor a survey of where the field stands in terms of scientific progress and what its resources for research have been, are now, and will likely be over the years immediately ahead, plus projections of the field's future needs. That survey forms the basis of much of the present discussion.

The resources for research in this field as in all others are mainly comprised of: financial support to cover the costs of research; highly trained professional personnel to direct and conduct the investigative effort; and appropriate institutional facilities where the research can be carried out. Of these resources, money, personnel and facilities, the most vital is money. That a significant and sustained infusion of funds will stimulate research activity in a special field has been repeatedly demonstrated. Attention in this chapter will therefore focus primarily on the monetary resources for research in this particular area of biomedical science.

FUNDING

Historic perspective

Virtually all of our present knowledge concerning the male and female reproductive systems has been gained during the past half century. The initiation of systematic studies in this area did not get underway until the mid-twenties. Support for these studies over the next two decades came primarily from local institutional funds and the pharmaceutical industry. A programme of supplementary aid initiated by the Rockefeller family in 1921 provided support averaging around $70 000 per year up to 1945.

The post World War II era witnessed the advent of US governmental support of health science research on a scale unparalleled in history. Although the ability to regulate reproductive performance is a major factor in determining maternal and child health, the reproductive sciences were almost totally excluded from this source of support for fifteen years, i.e. to 1960.

In the period between 1960 and 1965, mounting public concern over the rapidly expanding population forced the US government to alter its negative stance on support of reproductive research aimed at the control of human fertility. In 1963, the National Institute of Child Health and Human Development (NICHD) was established with a broad mandate that included funding of research in the reproductive sciences and family planning methods. However most of the funds were diverted to the study of early human development.

Fortunately such research did receive a welcome stimulus during this period by action on the part of private philanthropy, especially by the Ford Foundation. Thus, by 1965 the combined support of all US sources reached $31 million and represented 83.6% of worldwide support for research in this field.

The decade of growth and regression

Finally in 1968, public pressure forced creation of the Center for Population Research (CPR) within the NICHD, and thereupon support became available in sharply increasing amounts from the US government over the next half dozen years. During this same period, the total support made available for research in the reproductive sciences and contraceptive development by the United States, 15 other industrialized nations and nine developing countries or regions rose from a low of $31 million in 1965 to $119 million in 1974 (Table 1 and Figure 1). However, in terms of constant dollars (1970 = 100) this support reached a peak in 1973 and has since been declining due to the effect of inflation on the purchasing power of the dollar.

This current dwindling of support comes at a most inopportune time. Over the past few years great progress has been made in understanding the complex reproductive process, and the research enterprise has the professional and institutional capacity in hand to advance at an even more rapid pace.

The bulk of support for this field over the past decade has been coming from the United States. As indicated above, in 1965 this reached 83.6% of worldwide expenditures; by 1974 this had dropped to 68.3% (Table 1). Support from the 15 other developed nations surveyed doubled from 15.7 to 30.5% over the same period. Although there was little change in the percentage contributed by the developing nations during this period the amount in constant dollars quadrupled. The Ford survey team expressed the opinion that in the interests of a more equitable distribution of the responsibility for support of research in this field, contributions from the 15 other industrialized nations should be augmented to 40%. This, however, does not seem a likely prospect since the more affluent nations in this group have themselves no pressing population problems at home.

Notable changes also occurred during this 10-year period in the percentage of worldwide support provided by governmental agencies, philanthropy and industry. Most significantly the share from governmental sources rose sharply from 44.1% to 69.4%. This gain was accompanied by drastic declines in the percentage contributed by both philanthropy and industry (Table 2). The latter change reflects industry's growing disenchantment with the contraceptive field

Table 1 Total expenditures for research in the reproductive sciences and contraceptive development by country of origin, 1965, 1969–74 (current and constant US dollars in thousands, 1970 = 100)

*Country of origin**	*1965*	*1969*	*1970*	*1971*	*1972*	*1973*	*1974*
Total all countries							
Current dollars	31 022	54 546	71 462	94 483	110 224	117 430	118 723
Constant dollars	38 270	57 893	71 462	90 390	100 825	100 957	91 146
United States							
Current dollars	25 928	41 537	55 009	71 663	79 724	82 070	79 104
Constant dollars	32 010	44 188	55 009	68 906	73 819	71 991	62 287
Other industrialized countries (15)							
Current dollars	4 886	11 992	15 267	21 126	28 811	33 039	38 029
Constant dollars	5 992	12 634	15 267	19 908	25 505	27 093	27 771
Developing countries (9)							
Current dollars	208	1 017	1 186	1 694	1 689	2 321	1 590
Constant dollars	268	1 070	1 186	1 577	1 501	1 873	1 088
Percent distribution (based on constant US dollars)							
All countries	100.0	100.0	100.0	100.0	100.0	100.0	100.0
United States	83.6	76.4	77.0	76.3	72.4	69.9	68.3
Other industrialized countries	15.7	21.8	21.3	22.0	26.1	28.1	30.5
Developing countries	0.7	1.8	1.7	1.7	1.5	2.0	1.2

* *Countries:* United States; *Other Industrialized Countries:* Belgium, Britain, Canada, France, Germany, Israel, Japan, Italy, Netherlands, Australia, New Zealand, Scandinavian countries—Denmark, Finland, Norway and Sweden; *Developing Countries:* Egypt, Hong Kong, India, Philippines, Thailand, South Korea, Africa, Iran, Turkey.

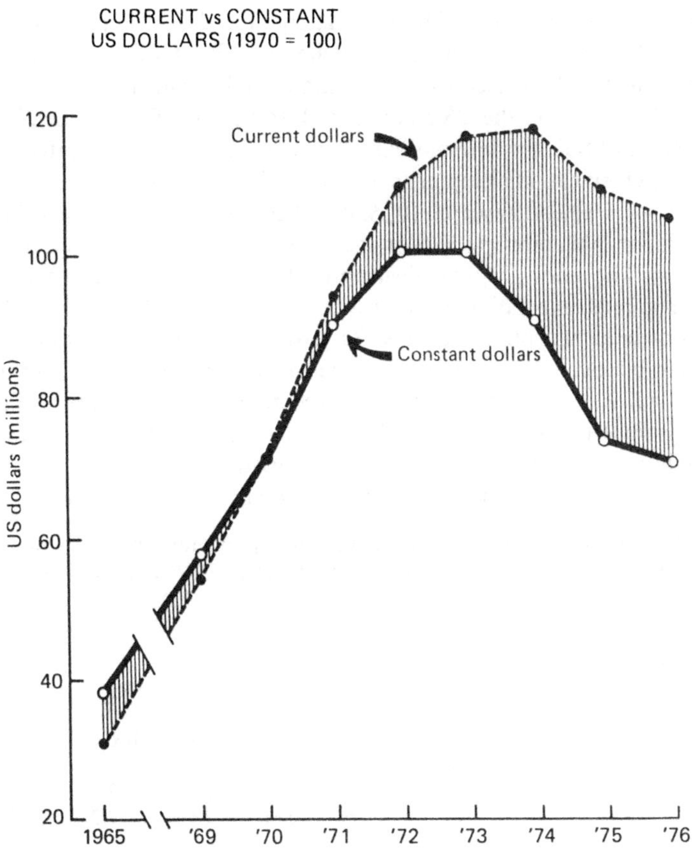

Figure 1 Worldwide expenditure for reproductive research

as a market area. This came about as a result of the imposition of regulations that have made the development of a new product a lengthier and more costly process – estimated at 10 years and $20 million. This is unfortunate because contraceptive development is appropriately and traditionally a function of industry.

In this connection, the past decade has witnessed the emergence of agencies in the public sector that are helping to fill the void left by the partial withdrawal of industry from the development, testing and distribution of new or improved contraceptive products. These agencies, collectively and loosely referred to as the Public Sector, include: the Population Council's International Committee for Contraception Research (ICCR); the World Health Organization's Special Programme of Research, Development and Research Training in Human Reproduction; United Nations Fund for Population Activities (UNFPA); the three contract branches of the CPR, i.e. Contraceptive Development, Contraceptive Evaluation and Behavioral Sciences; The Research Division of the US Agency for International Development's Office of Population (AID); the International Development Research Center of Canada (IDRC); Overseas Development Ministry (ODM) of Britain; and the Indian Council for Medical Research (ICMR). These agencies derive their funds from government, philanthropy and/or the several existing international assistance agencies. The contraceptive development activities of these agencies now involve annual expenditures of around $26 million. Although each agency operates independently and has its own particular programme, there is considerable overlap in the areas of their research interest. The contraceptive testing activities of these agencies generally involve some collaborative relationship with industry, especially for the supply of drugs or devices and the availability of compounds patented by industry. These agencies do not themselves have any manufacturing or retail distribution capabilities. The

Table 2 Percent distribution of expenditure for reproductive research and contraceptive development, by country and sector,* 1965 and 1969–74 (based on 1970 US dollars)

Country and sector	*1965*	*1969*	*1970*	*1971*	*1972*	*1973*	*1974*
All countries	100.0	100.0	100.0	100.0	100.0	100.0	100.0
Government	44.1	54.9	54.7	55.6	65.7	70.3	69.4
Philanthropy	21.8	19.5	24.3	25.5	17.1	14.4	14.2
Industry	34.1	25.6	21.0	18.9	17.2	15.3	16.4
United States	100.0	100.0	100.0	100.0	100.0	100.0	100.0
Government	35.7	45.1	46.0	46.5	58.6	61.9	61.0
Philanthropy	25.5	25.0	30.5	32.8	22.9	19.7	20.3
Industry	38.8	29.9	23.5	20.7	18.6	18.4	18.7
Developed countries	100.0	100.0	100.0	100.0	100.0	100.0	100.0
Government	86.4	85.4	82.7	83.9	84.0	90.4	87.1
Philanthropy	3.1	2.0	3.6	2.2	1.6	1.5	1.1
Industry	10.4	12.6	13.7	13.9	14.4	8.1	11.8
Developing countries	100.0	100.0	100.0	100.0	100.0	100.0	100.0
Government	97.0	98.5	98.8	98.8	99.1	98.9	98.8
Philanthropy	0.0	0.5	0.0	0.3	0.0	0.4	0.0
Industry	3.0	1.0	1.2	0.9	0.9	0.7	1.2

* See footnote, Table 1.
Note: Percentages may not add to 100 because of rounding.

CPR, ICCR and WHO are currently sponsoring major programmes in the premarket testing of new or improved contraceptive modalities. Ultimately, however, the manufacture and distribution of any approved product must in most instances be done by industry through licensing arrangements that guarantee low cost distribution to low income areas.

Lest it appear that an annual expenditure in excess of $100 million for sex-related research is reasonably adequate, cognizance should be taken of the fact that this does not compare favourably with the support given to other high priority fields in health-related research, and constitutes only a miniscule part of the expenditures for all medical research or for international assistance where family planning is a key element in attaining a beneficial outcome. In 1974, expenditures by the US government for reproductive research constituted only 1.6% of its allocations for medical research. Even more inexplicable is the observation that the world's international assistance agencies spent only 0.2% of their funds for such research in that year. Clearly research having the control of human fertility as its objective is not perceived as an urgent matter by any nation with the possible exception of China whose expenditures for such research are not available.

Funding outlook and projected needs

When the Ford survey was completed, anticipated increases in funding were nowhere to be found. Cutbacks had already become nearly universal, and estimates of worldwide funding in the years ahead showed anticipated reductions. These have become realities and the downward trend continues although not so much in real dollars as in constant dollars.

Since the US government accounts for nearly half of the world's support for this field, and most of this is channelled through the CPR, the level of funding by that agency in constant dollars serves as a rough guide to support for the field at large. Support by the CPR has not diminished over the past three years, but as a result of the spiralling costs of research and inflationary trends these funds support less and less research. This is made evident by the serious decline in the number of approved grant applications that can be funded; this had reached 50% in 1969 and by 1977 had dipped to one in four, or 25%! This slackening of research activity has been further accentuated by the severe cutbacks in support by philanthropy and industry. One small ray of promise stems from a modest increase in funds appropriated for the CPR in 1978. Motivation for that increase was the expressed hope that better means of contraception would lessen the need for abortion. Total NIH expenditures for reproductive research in 1978 are expected to approximate 3% of expenditures for medical research.

There is no accurate determinant of the adequacy of funding, but there are some indicators of inadequacy such as inability to fund meritorious projects and the uneven level of funding in the reproductive field *vis-à-vis* other fields in the health area. The Ford survey team estimated that simply to maintain the 1974 level of activity ($119 million) would require, as a result of inflation, $197 million by 1980 (Table 3). At the other extreme, a projected priority of 10% of all expenditures for medical research would have raised the level of funding to $671 million by 1978 and $766 million in 1980. A more realistic projection of need based on an adequate exploitation of identified problem areas in the field called for a tripling of funding in 1976 rising to $530 million in 1978, and nearly one half billion in 1980. Considering that NIH is able to fund only one fourth of the approved grant applications, this projected tripling of the level of support is not unreasonable. Meeting this goal would require in 1978 a contribution of $291 million by the US, $133 million by the 15 other developed nations and $5.6 million by the developing nations. These funding targets are justified not only because of the urgent problems this field seeks to solve, but in order to exploit adequately the new knowledge of reproductive processes already in hand.

Table 3 Three levels of projected funding for reproductive research and contraceptive development, 1974–80 (in millions of current US dollars)*

Funding level	*1974 (actual)*	*1976*	*1977*	*1978*	*1979*	*1980*
Maintenance, 1974 level	118.7	142.7	156.5	170.5	184.3	197.5
High priority †	472.6	566.0	619.7	671.8	721.8	766.3
Existing knowledge ‡	na	360.5	395.2	430.3	464.8	497.6
United States	na	246.2	269.2	291.1	311.3	328.1
Other developed countries	na	110.0	121.1	133.6	147.2	162.3
Developing countries	na	4.3	4.9	5.6	6.3	7.2

* Inflation factors for the United States derived from H. B. Woolley; for other nations, factors are based on extrapolation to 1980 of the average annual rate of increase in consumer price indices for 1969–74.

† This is 10% of medical research expenditures.

‡ To take adequate advantage of existing knowledge and opportunities, the distribution assumes that the proportion of total funds for the field in 1974 from the United States (68.3%), other developed countries (30.5%) and developing countries (1.2%) will be the same in 1976 and will change in subsequent years only as a result of differential rates of inflation.

Note: na = not applicable.

From Koblinsky, Jaffe and Greer (1976)

PROFESSIONAL PERSONNEL AND FACILITIES

The number of professional people engaged in research on reproduction and contraceptive development can only be estimated. From a variety of data sources, the Ford survey team concluded that there can be no less than 2500 and probably no more than 3000 individuals devoting a significant portion of their time and effort to research in this area. The survey also identified 419 institutions where research of this nature is in progress. Of these, 176 were in the US, 162 in the other 15 industrialized nations surveyed, and an estimated 20 in Latin America where firm data were not forthcoming.

Information concerning the geographical location of investigative activity, as revealed by numbers of papers published in internationally recognized journals, was provided by the Reproduction Research Information Service. Of the 45 060 papers published between 1970 and 1975, 92% originated from the developed world with North America and Western Europe accounting for 83%. The 8% coming from the developing countries is not a fair measure of investigative activity in that part of the world, since much of the work done there is of clinical nature and more likely to appear in journals having local circulation.

THE ADVANTAGES AND DISADVANTAGES OF CONDUCTING RESEARCH IN THE DEVELOPING *VIS-À-VIS* THE DEVELOPED NATIONS

Obviously there is a great imbalance in availability of funds for, and the extent of, research activity between the developed and the developing countries. This is in large part due to the logistic difficulties inherent in the pursuit of research in the less industrialized nations. Among these is the usual necessity of obtaining support from outside the home country; the fact that most equipment must be imported and repair service is often lacking; standardized laboratory animals and animal foods are often not available; the same holds for air-conditioned quarters; and competent assistance for highly technical research is generally in short supply. Despite these odds, many third world investigators have amply demonstrated that they can conduct research of the highest quality. They deserve encouragement and greater opportunities for the exercise of their talents which are the equal of those anywhere in the world. These needs are especially great in respect to fundamental research, which should be expanded in those areas where many able and well-trained scientists are being denied opportunities for intellectual fulfilment and the satisfaction of competing with investigators in the developed nations on a fair and equal basis. The tendency to perceive the role of third world investigators as limited to clinical studies, especially the testing of new or improved contraceptives, is all too prevalent.

Third world scientists, basic and clinical investigators alike, do have some distinct advantages. One is the opportunity of studying contraceptives under field conditions. There also the development of a contraceptive can be followed by the same investigator from inception to application. This is an advantage that is largely denied to investigators in many of the most highly industrialized nations where regulatory restrictions regarding the use of human subjects are definitely prohibitive. They also have the advantage of being directly and intimately acquainted with any special contraceptive needs that their own people may have and can direct their studies accordingly.

CONCLUSIONS

It is abundantly evident that: (1) increased support of research on reproduction and human fertility control is a matter of critical importance to the future welfare of humankind; (2) the mounting of a strong programme of research in this area was handicapped and delayed for nearly half a century by social, cultural and religious taboos and political sensitivity; (3) over the past 15 years reproductive research has undergone rapid expansion and made great progress concomitant with the availability of significantly increased financial support; (4) no further intensification of effort in this field can be achieved unless and until the necessary funds are made available; (5) the amount of money required for the development of an adequate effort in this field is of such magnitude that it can only be provided by government as the primary source; (6) if additional support is not forthcoming soon this field will gradually lose the talent and momentum it has so recently gained; and (7) at present this field remains poised as never before to advance at an even more rapid pace, and capitalize on the gains made in wide-ranging studies aimed at better understanding of the complex reproductive process and improved means of human conception control.

Bibliography

Greep, R. O., Koblinsky, M. A. and Jaffe, F. S. (1976). *Reproduction and Human Welfare: A Challenge to Research.* (Cambridge: MIT Press). Summarized in *Bioscience,* **26,** 677

Greep, R. O. and Koblinsky, M. A. (1977). *Frontiers in Reproduction and Fertility Control.* (Cambridge, Mass.: MIT Press)

Koblinsky, M. A., Jaffe, F. S. and Greep, R. O. (1976). Funding for reproduction research: The status and the needs. *Family Planning Perspectives,* **8,** 212

16

Resources for programmes

Nafis Sadik

INTRODUCTION	266
HUMAN RIGHTS	266
STRATEGIES FOR PROGRESS	266
ROLE OF UNFPA	267
Planning for the future	268
UNMET NEEDS	269
PRESENT POPULATION STATUS	269
DEMAND FOR RESOURCES	270
Availability of family planning	271
FUTURE TRENDS	271

INTRODUCTION

Twenty-one years ago, before the United Nations Fund for Population Activities came into existence, the Food and Agriculture Organization held its ninth conference. Professor Arnold Toynbee gave a speech on population and food supply. This was years before any multilateral, bilateral or even non-governmental organizations and agencies had initiated population assistance programmes; in fact, almost before there was any recognition – or at least enough recognition – of the population situation of the world.

Professor Toynbee at that time raised the question as to what is the true end of man: 'Is it to populate the earth with the maximum number of human beings or is it to enable human beings to lead the best kind of life . . . ?' He gave the answer that 'living human beings, whatever their number, shall develop the highest capacities of their nature . . . and what we should aim at is the optimum size population for this purpose in the economic and social circumstances of each succeeding generation'.

HUMAN RIGHTS

Much has happened in the world since that statement. Progress, although some of it is not as rapid as many of us might have wished, has taken place on many fronts to achieve for the world's peoples the rights guaranteed to everyone in international instruments and in legal utterances at various conventions and conferences held under United Nations auspices. There is the Universal Declaration of Human Rights, the Declaration of the Rights of the Child, the International Covenant on Economic, Social and Cultural Rights, the World Population Plan of Action, the World Plan of Action for the Implementation of Objectives of the International Women's Year, and more recently, the Declaration of Alma Ata on Primary Health Care.

The human rights defined in these and other international declarations and covenants are fundamental freedoms for all of us. So long as one person is denied his or her right to a standard of living adequate for the health and wellbeing of his or her family, including food, clothing, employment, housing, medical care and social services, the right to information and services to plan the size and the number and the spacing of children, and the right to security, none of us is free.

STRATEGIES FOR PROGRESS

Since that historic FAO Conference of 21 years ago, there has been worldwide recognition of the intimate relationship between and among the various elements that, taken together, constitute socio-economic development. This is particularly true of the relationship between population and socio-economic development.

In sectors where social change or social-attitude change is a fundamental requirement for acceptance of any development process, it has become very clear that a strategy regarding population growth cannot be treated in isolation, apart from a strategy for employment or education or industrialization and so on. Together, any international or nationally adopted strategies for national or international progress must be considered as components of a total system.

This fact of international life has generally been recognized in a number of internationally adopted instruments and strategies designed to map a world-wide attack on the world's problems. For example, the World Population Plan of Action, adopted at the 1974 World Population Conference in Bucharest by consensus of 135 states, points out that

> 'the basis for an effective solution of population problems is, above all, socio-economic transformation. A population policy may have a certain success if it constitutes an integral part of socio-economic development; its contribution to the solution of world development problems is hence only partial, as is the case with other sectoral strategies. Consequently, the Plan of Action must be considered as an important component of the system of international strategies and as an instrument of the international community for the promotion of economic development, quality of life, human rights and fundamental freedoms'.

Yet, at the World Food Conference which took place later in the same year it required a major effort to include any reference to the relationship between population and food. In fact, the Conference did not wish to mention the word 'population' at all because it felt it would be controversial. The same has been true of discussions concerning the new international economic order.

ROLE OF UNFPA

The United Nations Fund for Population Activities has recognized the close relationship between population, food, employment and other aspects of socio-economic life from the time it became operational in 1969. As a Fund of the General Assembly, the United Nations Fund for Population Activities works closely with the Food and Agriculture Organization, the World Health Organization, the International Labour Organization, the United Nations

Educational, Scientific and Cultural Organization, the United Nations Children's Fund, and so on.

The Fund's mandate from the United Nations Economic and Social Council includes the promotion of awareness 'of the social, economic and environmental implications of national and international population problems; of the human rights aspects of family planning; and of possible strategies to deal with them in accordance with the plans and priorities of each country . . .'.

That the Fund has been somewhat successful in doing the job it has been mandated to do is reflected in the fact that the United Nations Fund for Population Activities has grown from a small fund of less than $3 million in 1969 to become the largest multilateral funding source for population assistance, with cumulative resources of over $500 million pledged by 93 countries, with a global programme under which the Fund has implemented more than 1900 population projects in assisting 114 developing countries throughout the world.

Of the 93 contributing countries, there are ten major donors, of which the United States is the largest donor and which has pledged $28 million in 1978. The other nine are Japan and the developed countries of Western Europe. The Fund's contributors include pledges from the Arab oil-rich countries which have contributed about $12 million. The remainder of the contributions come from the developing countries themselves.

Planning for the future

Many of the projects that developing countries ask us to fund – population, housing and agricultural censuses; maternal and child health-based family planning programmes, which include in many cases nutritional education and disease control programmes; communication and information programmes; fertility surveys and so on – assist development planners enormously in current planning and in planning for the future.

Such planning must include infants, young children and pregnant and lactating mothers who constitute a large proportion of the population in most developing countries. If one takes into account the fact that over 40% of the population in many countries is under 12 years of age, then in fact women and children constitute the majority; three-quarters of the population of many developing countries are women and children. The Fund feels that maternal and child health/family planning programmes are one of the most important elements of any health or development activity. Such activities aim to reduce rates of mortality and morbidity and are often the beginning of the demographic transition from high to low death and birth rates. The largest share of the Fund's total budget (over 60%) goes to providing assistance for family planning programmes.

Interest in migratory movements, which increasingly is a kind of programme for which our assistance is now being requested, is being evidenced by developing countries, since migration not only affects demand but also employment, housing, the processing, marketing and distribution of food, etc.

UNMET NEEDS

Those of us in the population field have a great opportunity for collaboration in a number of areas that can help to spell progress for the world's people – in the area of rural development, in land settlement and resettlement, in increasing the employment and status of women (and this is a subject which needs a great deal more attention than has been given to it), in educating and motivating people to move from crowded urban areas to satellite cities, to name just a few.

Whatever we do, we must not lose sight of the fact that when we use such terms as 'population' or 'food' or 'employment', we are not talking in generalities, we are talking about people.

We are talking about two-thirds of the world's people who lack the basic requirements for food, for shelter, for education, for health, for jobs, and for all of the other necessities that most other people in developed countries take for granted.

We are talking about the more than 15 million children under the age of 5 who die each year of the combined effects of malnutrition and infection.

We are talking about the hundreds of millions whose food and diet deficiencies reduce their productivities, their alertness, their endurance and their development.

We are also talking about the millions of children who are brain-damaged or retarded because of prenatal and infant malnutrition.

Sometimes it appears that the spectres of hunger, ill-health, unemployment and so on are like figures on a treadmill chasing but never catching each other, while the treadmill itself seems to go faster and faster. For even in those countries where caloric intake and nutritional standards may be adequate today, they may not, because of population growth, be adequate for tomorrow's population.

PRESENT POPULATION STATUS

Recently, the United Nations conducted a survey, called the Third Population

Inquiry, of the member nations of the United Nations. As a result of the Inquiry, the United Nations has revised its population estimates. Although the global growth rate has remained steady at about 1.9% a year, the United Nations revised downwards its estimates of the number of people at present on the planet and forecast a slowing-down rate of growth in all areas of the world.

That population factors are now almost a universally accepted element of development policy in developing countries can be seen in the increasing emphasis given to population. A complementary United Nations survey to the Third Population Inquiry, also taken during 1976, pointed out some interesting facts in this regard, as follows:

* Out of 114 developing countries 83 have entrusted a central planning authority with the task of integrating population factors with development planning.
* Sixty-nine countries believe that the current rate of natural population increase imposes severe constraints on the attainment of development objectives.
* Out of the 114 developing countries surveyed 63% are concerned with some aspect of their demographic situation – internal migration, morbidity and mortality, the current rate of national population increase, international migration and so on.
* Fifty-four developing countries consider that their rates of fertility are too high. Of these, 18 are in Asia, 18 in Africa, 16 in Latin America and two in the Middle East, and together they comprise 82% of the population in the developing world.
* Eighty-two governments themselves provide either direct or indirect support to fertility regulation measures, regardless of their own policies on natural increase and national fertility.
* Only eight of the 114 developing countries surveyed deny access to the use of modern methods of fertility regulation.
* Ninety-five countries consider that their population distribution is either substantially or extremely unacceptable.
* Seventy-nine countries view their levels of morbidity and mortality as a problem.

DEMAND FOR RESOURCES

From the vantage point of the United Nations Fund for Population Activities, I would like to point out that requests for assistance in the field of population now far outstrip our resources. Even though this year our resources will total about $100 million, the requests for assistance that we have on hand are much greater. Most of these requests are from countries which wish to initiate or expand family planning programmes.

All of the Asian countries have such programmes, most of which are aimed at reducing rates of growth. But now such family planning programmes are also being conducted in many Latin American countries as well, including Mexico, Chile, the Dominican Republic, etc. Recently, Brazil also agreed that its population must have family planning as a basic human right and is now taking steps to provide services.

In Africa, many countries now completing their first censuses are looking at their population policies. Many of them feel that their rates of growth and their fertility levels are too high, although, on the other hand, some also feel that their fertility levels are too low and must be increased.

Availability of family planning

While there has been a general decline in the fertility around the world – and this trend may be expected to continue according to demographers – surveys indicate that availability and accessibility of family planning information and supplies is a real problem for rural populations and for urban poor. The proper distribution of services and the accessibility of these social services is, of course, fundamental not only to family planning programmes but to the provision of all services in developing countries.

A number of measures, therefore, need to be undertaken including urging that all governments provide the necessary technology to all of its people in the best possible manner, integrating family planning concepts into all community activities, encouraging greater involvement of women in the decision-making and policy-making process, and looking at the future education of and catering to the needs of the young population.

FUTURE TRENDS

Trends today do not allow room for complacency, however, particularly when we remember that a global rate of growth of 1.9% means that the world's population will double in about 37 years, and when we remember that in the developing world where two-thirds of the world's population lives, the doubling time is even shorter, about 25 years, because the average rate of growth in the developing countries is 2.6%. The most likely outcome of the present trend, therefore, is that the world's population will stabilize at about three times its present level, that is to say, at 12 billion nearly a century from now – assuming a constantly falling rate of fertility.

Those of us in the population field should not be discouraged about the world of the future. Rather, we should remember the statement in the World Population Plan of Action: 'Of all things in the world, people are the most precious. Man's knowledge and ability to master himself and his environment will continue to grow. Mankind's future can be made infinitely bright'.

SECTION FOUR

Conclusions

Fertility regulation has many aspects, from breast feeding to induced abortion. Modern techniques of family planning are an essential and wanted addition to traditional methods. Societies benefit from access to the fullest possible range of methods. Broader policies and improved management promises more rapid, large scale and immediate extension of family planning services than the development and introduction of new methods of contraception.

Successful programmes build on community resources and can be used as an element in other aspects of community development.

Family planning has come a long way in the past decade. The structure of successful programmes is increasingly well understood. The effort now must be to apply this knowledge for the benefit of hundreds of millions of couples who are still beyond choice when it comes to child bearing.

17

Conclusions

Malcolm Potts
and
Pouru Bhiwandiwala

INTRODUCTION 276

THE TOTAL PICTURE 276

WHY DO SOME PROGRAMMES SUCCEED? 277

Promotion 277

Range of methods 279

Evolution of services 280

Community involvement 281

Self-sufficiency 282

Management 283

WHO DOES WHAT? 283

RESOURCES 285

THE PRESENCE OF ABORTION 288

THE POPULARITY OF STERILIZATION 289

FUTURE AND PRESENT METHODS 291

DEMAND AND SERVICES 294

CHOICE 296

INTRODUCTION

Family planning as a discipline has a brief history. Yet it is concerned with one of the fundamental problems of the twentieth century. Not surprisingly, there have been rapid changes and sometimes alternations of position and opinion. Many of the details of the subject have been disputed. But behind the academic debates, the bureaucratic quarrels and political disagreements, some major concepts have emerged and are agreed upon.

There is a broad relationship between incomes, urbanization, the opportunity for women to work, a number of lesser factors and a declining birth-rate. One way of expressing the explicit or implied aims of many family planning programmes in the developing world is to accelerate the trend towards lower fertility attendant on modernization. In some cases, an attempt is made to short-circuit it. The examples given in this volume suggest that this change can indeed take place.

But what of the 250 million couples who are estimated as being beyond the reach of family planning services? What do they do at present; are they totally without choice? What can be learnt from the previous experience of successful programmes? How can local schemes be replicated on a national scale? How should donor agencies distribute their resources to achieve the maximum effect? What are the relative roles of governmental and non-governmental agencies? Will new methods of fertility regulation make the task easier?

THE TOTAL PICTURE

Couples who do not use modern methods of family planning may still be taking some steps to control their fertility. In the past, family planning programmes often ignored this fact, but the real need is to understand and capitalize on traditional practices. It is useful in family planning to attempt to see the total complex of factors which affect achieved family size, because the elements which fall within a family planning programme are never the sole factors. Some government family planning programmes only influence a minority of the factors controlling human fertility. In Sri Lanka, a rising age of marriage over the past ten years has played a greater role in the decline in the birth-rate than the national family planning programme. In many developing countries, more births are averted by breast feeding than by the existing family planning services. To return to the Sri Lankan example, breast feeding plays a bigger role in fertility control than sterilization and modern contraception. The cost of importing infant formulas for the relatively small numbers who have abandoned this practice already exceeds the amount of overseas money provided by all the external family planning organizations active in the country. If half the women now breast feeding were to turn to bottle feeding, the cost of importing the necessary infant formulas would exceed the budget of the Health Ministry.

In some countries, *coitus interruptus* (male withdrawal) could have been singled out for discussion as much as breast feeding. To complete the Sri Lankan example, for every woman or man using a 'modern method' of family planning in 1975, there was another using a traditional method such as the rhythm method or *coitus interruptus*. In Turkey, the use of *coitus interruptus* has remained ahead of modern methods over the past decade.

The use of a method of limited duration (such as lactation), or of one with what may be a higher failure rate (such as *coitus interruptus*) by a great many people is more important for population change than highly predictable, sophisticated methods used by a few. There is nothing contradictory about an administrator trying to launch an advertising campaign to promote breast feeding, and an individual family planning worker advising a mother who may be seeking advice early in lactation, to adopt a modern method of family planning soon. By seeking specialized advice, an individual may prove to be an exception; in planning programmes we must also think of those who do not use, or cannot reach, formal services.

WHY DO SOME PROGRAMMES SUCCEED?

Proven successes and promising family planning programmes involve only a small proportion of those that have been initiated. For every successful programme there are a number that have failed. Whenever success is irregularly distributed, it is reasonable to ask whether it is because some societies are more receptive than others to choices in fertility regulation, or whether common characteristics can be identified in the successful programmes which are attempting to meet the same basic needs among potential recipients.

The hypothesis set out in this volume is that it is often barriers on the side of the provider which account for the irregular outcome of many programmes. It may be suggested that many of the major issues in family planning do not revolve around the problems of motivating couples or supplying family planning services to villages or urban slums, but are mainly matters of political policy setting and programme management.

Promotion

Obviously, motivation is important and will be dealt with first, before turning to other more difficult issues. When the experience of successful programmes from a wide range of countries is assembled, the assumed problem of major cultural differences between communities often largely dissolves, and the common problem which faces the poor in coping with a difficult and uncertain world surfaces as a uniting theme.

All family planning activities involve an important element of promotion. Even the mere availability of contraceptives, as the experience of Thai villages and Bombay railway stations (Chapters 5 and 7) shows, stimulates discussion and transmits an idea as well as the possibility of use. In many programmes, service needs outrun the available resources. In such a situation, promotion must take second place in the broad balance between services and promotion. However, while the emphasis of this volume is on services, this should not be taken as downgrading the significance of promotion. Clearly, availability must precede or occur in parallel with promotion. To propagate an idea which could not be implemented would be self-defeating. At the same time, the successful programmes reported have used a variety of colourful information and educational efforts. In general, successful programmes promote the idea of family planning rather than particular methods, although clear instruction and honest information about methods is essential. The experience of defining and promoting a particular brand image has been a key element in successful social marketing programmes (Chapter 8). Social marketing programmes have also demonstrated that local advertising agencies will handle contraceptive promotion as easily as they take on another account for a soap manufacturer.

A wide range of promotional techniques can be used. Indeed, it is almost impossible to find an everyday thing that cannot be brought in, in one form or another, to assist the cause of family planning. For example, the packaging of soups, sanitary napkins, infant feeding formulas and T-shirts can all carry family planning slogans, or coupons promoting or simplifying access to family planning. Even children's games, similar to Snakes and Ladders, have been modified so that the winner is the one gaining the most points for taking the steps that lead to the best control of human reproduction. On some occasions, it is possible to piggy-back messages at no cost. In one country, everybody who is vasectomized is given a free lottery ticket and in some areas has a chance to win a motorcycle.

Experienced administrators of successful programmes all take care to establish good relationships with the media. This not only helps to propagate family planning messages, but assists in pre-empting the spread of adverse rumours or misunderstandings. Maximum use is always made of satisfied clients and genuine side-effects are approached with maturity and honesty. People usually understand that anything which is widely used may occasionally have side-effects. In one fishing community it is pointed out that, *although shrimps are very tasty and good to eat, they can sometimes give people a rash* – a parallel that is applicable in human and biological terms to some contraceptive side-effects.

As a policy, it seems most appropriate that the technical assistance relevant to family planning promotion should come from within the country concerned. When the country itself cannot provide the necessary technical resources, these can be more appropriately drawn from a regional rather than a global level. In every community it is important to communicate using a vocabulary and metaphors that local people will understand and relate to. For example, one of the verbal analogies given by village family planning workers in Thailand is *'space your children like rubber trees, even your legs are apart'*.

The controversial history of family planning has made many people involved in the subject forget that it is related to human sexual activity, which is itself not very far removed from the more humorous aspects of human life. Coloured condoms have proved easier to distribute than plain ones. In Sweden, the promotion of condoms has been partly based on humour.

The short-term beneficial aspects of certain family planning methods have been largely overlooked. The fact that the Pill reduces menstrual blood loss is important, particularly in communities where women are often malnourished and anaemia is almost universal. As an example of the combination of the humorous and supposedly beneficial, the point has sometimes been made in the Orient that use of oral contraceptives can lead to a slight enlargement of the breasts – which is rarely regarded as a disadvantage. Another slightly earthy example comes from the promotional information associated with one particular spermicide (Neosampoon). Like most spermicides, it can cause mild irritation of the vaginal epithelium in addition to killing sperms. Advertising literature capitalizes on this, proclaiming *'Use Neosampoon for that warm sensation'*.

Briefly, the promotional aspect of family planning is important but also increasingly well understood. Tried and tested means of promoting any low-cost high-volume domestic item are applicable to contraceptives. It is in the freedom to use established channels or even to advertise contraceptives at all, that most limitations are found.

Range of methods

Successful programmes attempt to make a variety of fertility regulation options available, and successful programme managers are characterized by an enthusiastic ability to make the most of the limited methods available to them.

The need for breadth of choice was emphasized by the Tokyo Symposium. At the present time, many existing methods are arbitrarily excluded from entire countries by accidents of history, national laws or by the domestic policies of donor agencies. In India, oral contraceptives have never been used in the government family planning programmes, although they are the major element in neighbouring Malaysia and Thailand. When they have been made available through non-government initiative to poor populations, they have been eagerly received (Chapter 5). In Japan, where legal abortion has been available since 1949, intrauterine devices were only officially approved in the 1970s; oral contraceptives were used by few women and then supposedly to regulate their menstrual cycles. In Sweden, there is a tradition of liberal attitudes towards sex education, aggressive and amusing advertisements of condoms, and ready availability of the Pill and intrauterine devices; however, male sterilization was not available until a few years ago. From the point of view of the individual attempting to control their fertility, these paradoxes can prove expensive and destructive. Prior to the reform of the abortion laws in Britain in 1967, women wishing for termination of pregnancy, and who could afford it, would fly to Stockholm to solve their problems. Ten years later, Swedish men were flying to London to obtain a vasectomy. To underscore this same paradox, in neighbouring Eire (Southern Ireland), where the advertisement and sale of any method of contraception is totally illegal and where therapeutic abortion is unthinkable, it has proved possible to offer vasectomy for the simple reason that nobody had remembered to pass a law against it! Therefore, it is possible to have a situation where a man is not able to purchase a condom, his wife cannot obtain a sterilization because of policies within hospitals, an abortion would be illegal and yet vasectomy can be made available.

The desire to use as wide a range of methods as possible is a common factor uniting the work of those who have implemented successful programmes. The most acceptable and cost-effective programmes can only be achieved if a full range of methods can be used. It is interesting to speculate how the successful and sensitive Japanese Family Planning Association (Chapter 9) would have handled Pills had they been available. The receptivity of village communities to sterilization seems as great in Indonesia (where it is partially excluded from the government programme) as in Sri Lanka or Thailand (where it is part of the programme). In practice, where programme managers find themselves restricted to one or two methods, they will do the best they can and if, in extreme circumstances, a method in current use were to be suddenly denied them, no doubt they would find a substitute.

Evolution of services

Fortunately the developing world is moving to wider family planning options more rapidly than did the West. As has been pointed out, the evolution of family planning services usually follows a predictable course, moving from doctor-staffed, clinic-based facilities offering the reversible methods of contraception, on to the surgical options and finally dealing with the problem of abortion. Observation suggests that countries go through these evolutionary steps with increasing rapidity. Policies which took more than a generation to develop in Britain or the United States have been achieved in a decade or less in some developing countries. For example, Margaret Sanger in the USA and Marie Stopes in the United Kingdom opened the first family planning clinics in the 1920s, and the world's first clinic was set up in Holland in the 19th century. Yet it was not until the 1950s that male and female sterilization became available in the United States as a realistic option, and it was only in 1974 that the US Supreme Court struck down laws restricting abortion services. In the Philippines, the importation of contraceptives was illegal until the late 1960s; a government programme beginning in clinics and then extending into the community for the reversible methods of contraception evolved rapidly in the early 1970s; and by 1975 male and female sterilization were becoming an option and are now a major part of the programme. The evidence is that Mexico, which has begun to set national policies in family planning even more recently, may go through the same evolution at a more accelerated pace.

Community involvement

Most successful programmes entail considerable community involvement – whether through the ancient *banjar* system in Bali (Chapter 4), the *Zilla Parishads* in Maharashtra (Chapter 7) or the newly trained village contraceptive distributors in Thailand (Chapter 5), Brazil or Colombia. In the last analysis, the only people available to the poor are often the poor themselves.

The Tokyo Symposium emphasized the theme of carrying decision-making and responsibility for services nearer to the community, and this concept is being increasingly appreciated in several aspects of socio-economic development. One of the most encouraging features common to successful family planning programmes is not only the involvement of the community, but the capacity, commitment and ingenuity of the community in helping to solve its own problems.

But, at some stage professional groups do have to offer some additional input, however small, into the community. In Thailand skilled teams move across the country, district by district, selecting and training key staff and leaving behind a usable network which requires relatively less input to sustain than to set up. In Howrah, seven hand-picked centres were used to train workers for the next 50 centres who, in turn, trained more personnel for 203 centres (Chapter 6). In Maharashtra, an effort is made to build on the governmental infrastructure of subcentres for health. Whether as a wave that breaks over the countryside, or as a multiplication like an amoeba that reproduces itself, rapid reliable replication of community-related family planning services has proven possible.

One limitation which some might have foreseen has not applied. In situations where educational opportunities have often been limited, the length of schooling has not been shown to be relevant to an adult's capacity to help his or her neighbours. In Calcutta, individuals with grade 8 to 10 education have proved *better* workers than those with higher education. In Taiwan, one of the most effective motivators proved to be a woman who was so intelligent that she was able to deceive the selection process into thinking she was literate (literacy was required of field workers), when in fact she could not read or write and had merely learnt what was for her a meaningless jumble of symbols.

Self-sufficiency

Any family planning programme may provide free services, subsidize the distribution (social marketing) of contraceptives and surgical services, provide family planning at cost or make a commercial profit. There is no reason why, in a developing society, all four options should not exist side by side. Certainly, there should be no antagonism among different systems.

The themes of community involvement and self-sufficiency come together in a happy combination. In a developing country with a weak infrastructure, the problem of organizing and paying the large number of field workers likely to be involved in family planning programmes can be a formidable one and corruption is not unknown. One solution is to ensure that the person closest to the community is receiving whatever financial reward is appropriate for the work from the subsidized sale of contraceptives, rather than from a central budget. An evaluation of a community-based service in Latin America recently demonstrated that in a group of villages, where the distributor was permitted to sell Pills and condoms for an agreed price, the consumer was actually paying *less* than in a control group of villages where the contraceptives were supposed to be free, but the distributor (for understandable human reasons) was making an illicit charge.

No nation wants to hold out the begging bowl. As countries develop, more and more of the population will be able to pay for family planning services, or governments will generate the revenue necessary to provide 'free' services. From the point of view of international donor agencies, the logical policy will be to shift an increasing proportion of the available budgets into commodity supplies and into the subsidy of surgical services. It is also predictable that the supply of contraceptives free of charge for developing nations to 'sell' in community-based distribution programmes is likely to persist longer than most other aspects of family planning aid. The budgetary policy of the US Agency for International Development with respect to family planning demonstrates such policies clearly (Figure 1).

Management

Finally, all successful programmes have business-like management, clear leadership and rational delegation of duties. There must be systematic attention to detail, as in Bali and Bombay. The freedom to hire and fire staff is an advantage private sector programmes have over governmental ones. It is notable that none of the programmes described earlier is subject to an excessive number of committees – a feature which has eroded the potential effectiveness of some programmes.

WHO DOES WHAT?

A major item in increasing the cost-effectiveness of any family planning programme revolves around the decisions concerning the use of paramedical workers. Experience shows that it is practical and responsible to remove the reversible methods of contraception from the direct supervision of physicians. A landmark policy in this field was set by the International Planned Parenthood Federation in 1973, and led to the validation and expansion of community-based family planning programmes in a number of countries. In 1976 an expert committee in the United Kingdom reviewed the problem of oral contraceptive distribution, and concluded that even in that country at a policy level it was reasonable to delegate the distribution of the Pill to trained and selected paramedical workers. Auxiliaries have been successfully involved in vasectomies, and in Bangladesh and Thailand nurse practitioners (in the case of Bangladesh, illiterate village women) have been taught female sterilization, which is the most demanding of all fertility regulation techniques.

In Africa, menstrual regulation is being successfully delegated to midwives. However, while it is increasingly recognized that paramedical workers must be involved in the reversible methods of contraception, in some developing countries and in nearly all urban areas, there is a sufficient reservoir of qualified doctors who are not currently involved in family planning. The experience of non-governmental organizations in involving such doctors and stimulating their work through financial rewards, which are the normal element in private practice, provides at least one way of recruiting the additional skills that are necessary (Chapter 7). The law (Chapter 14) is sometimes a factor which slows the process of delegation, even when there is objective evidence that it is responsible and creative to delegate specific tasks.

Figure 1 USAID population programme assistance

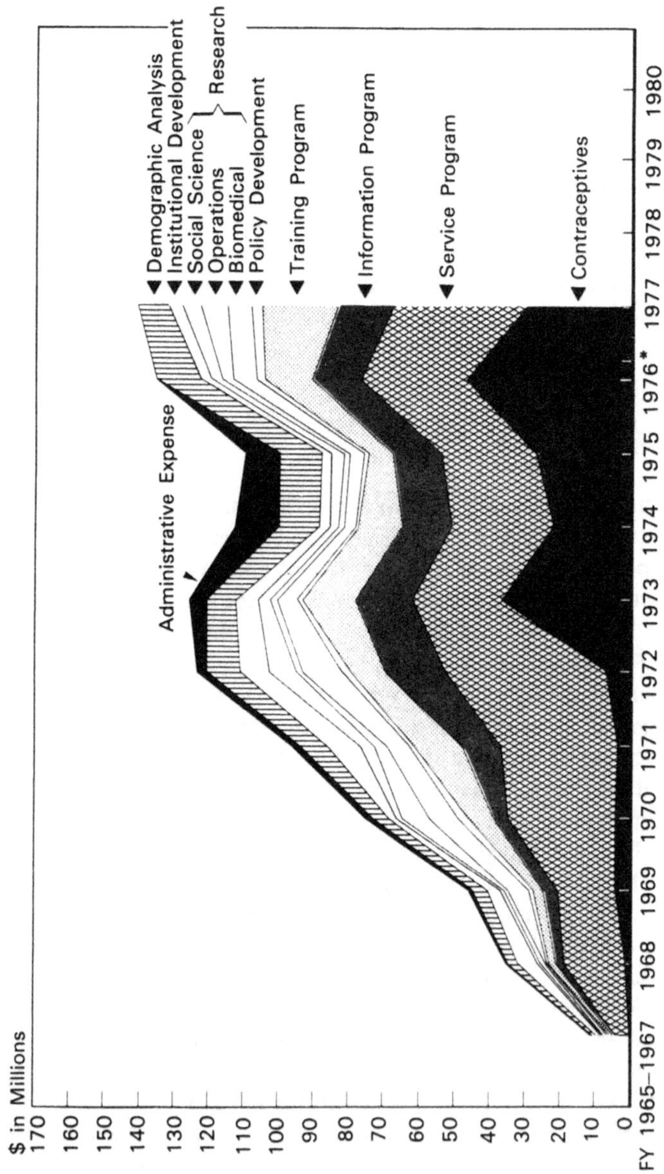

Financial Summary by Function FY 1965–1977 Obligations – in Millions of Dollars.

*Includes $7·3 millions contraceptive loan to Indonesia.

Conference quotations

"Housewives have the maturity, family life, experience and motivation to do an excellent job in field work."

"Some people must choose between half a kilo of sweet potatoes and a cycle of Pills."

"In a public institution they need three nurses to look after two patients, but in the private sector, one nurse will look after all the patients round the clock."

"Most funding agencies send you a man who tells you what you are doing is wrong, but does not tell you what to do."

"Not somebody from the capital who dresses differently, looks different, holds a cigarette differently, but someone they know and respect."

"They are experts in measuring failure but are unable to see success when it stares them in the face."

"Without government we are helpless. It is like a man and a woman – you need both."

"Nothing is free to the villagers – not even death."

"It is harder to get an American to eat with a spoon than to get a villager to use a contraceptive."

– Colombo, 1977 –

RESOURCES

The amount of money committed to family planning has grown enormously in the past decade. It is still not commensurate with the need and trivial in comparison to budgets set aside for defence, or even for other necessary aspects of development. However, as in the case of contraceptives, where the first need is to use what is available as effectively as possible, it must be admitted that there are now significant monies available for family planning

(Figure 2). The question must be asked continually as to how these resources are to be used to achieve the greatest effect and provide services to the millions of people who want to plan their families.

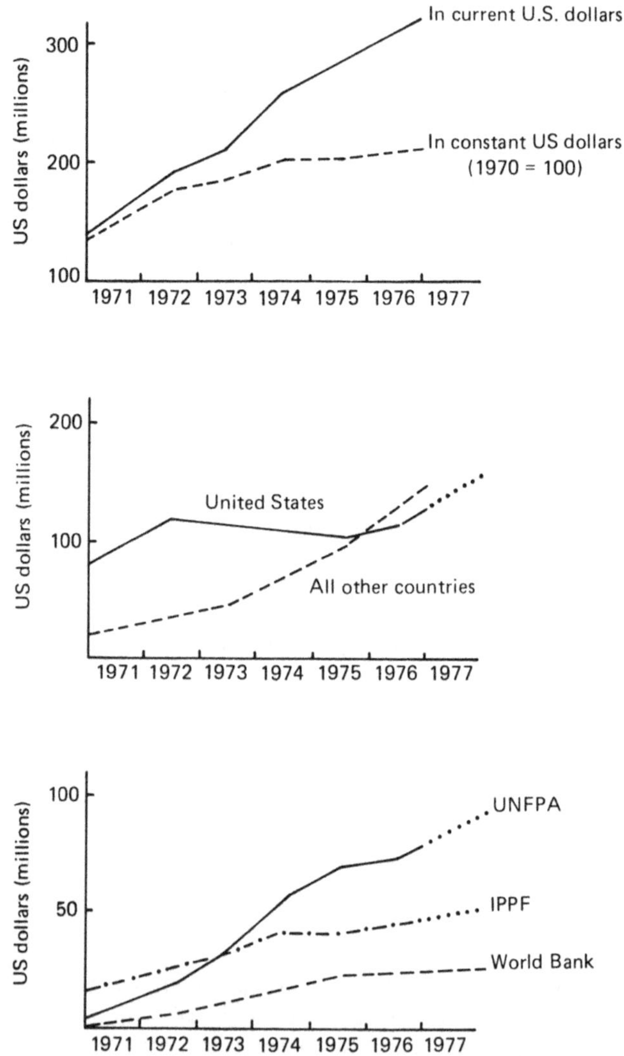

Figure 2 Total international population assistance (excluding double counting) 1971–77

Every resource has its own profile of constraints and areas where it has freedom of action. International governmental agencies, and industrialized countries which enter into bilateral aid programmes, usually have to wait until invited by the recipient government before they can extend support. This, for example, applies to the programme of loans which the World Bank has made relevant to family planning. However, because of the controversial nature of family planning, many countries arrive at the stage where the individuals who make up the government and the public would appreciate external assistance in relation to family planning, yet formal requests are not yet possible. Because of this unusual situation, which, for example, does not apply to agricultural development, a very important role has arisen for non-governmental agencies, of which the IPPF is the largest. Many of these receive considerable governmental contributions from Europe, North America and Japan and commonly carry out their work in close harmony at an informal level with the government of the recipient nation.

The smaller non-governmental organizations often pioneer the most controversial aspects of family planning. For example, the Association for Voluntary Sterilization in the United States has a long history and for most of its existence was considered a radical and frequently unpopular organization; yet today it manages a successful international project which is taking to developing countries the very services which were highly controversial in the United States for many years. On the whole, these more controversial activities have been supported from non-governmental contributions and, particularly, from private individuals and institutions in the United States of America. In a world of accelerating change and ever-increasing need for family planning, mechanisms need to be developed for bringing approprate amounts of governmental funding towards such organizations. USAID has found ways of beginning to do this, although European donor governments still have to face the problem.

Another emerging contribution of the non-governmental sector to family planning is in supporting and developing private services, which could then be taken up on a national scale to make a significant contribution to a country's family planning effort. For example, Population Services International, with non-governmental money, experimented in the social marketing of contraceptives. Then they received support from the IPPF (which is a non-governmental agency) to apply their experience in Sri Lanka, which has a population of only 14 million people. Subsequently they received governmental money to take the same experience to Bangladesh with a population of 84 million people. It is to be hoped that the sort of experience which has been reported in relation to privately managed surgical clinics may be supported in the same way (Chapter 7), so that a network of such clinics could be developed within a country. The evidence is that such clinics are a cost-effective way of providing services, and one which is acceptable to a significant segment of the community. Some of these private initiatives will require subsidy in very poor countries but, even then, will produce more service for the money invested than many existing models in this field.

Occasionally, a small input brings spectacular results. In one case, a single day's training in menstrual regulation by a visiting doctor and the supply of a few dollars' worth of equipment produced a service which performed 15 000 MRs in two years.*

THE PRESENCE OF ABORTION

While one or more family planning methods are often arbitrarily excluded in many family planning programmes, abortion is an element which is universally present wherever people attempt to control their fertility. Even where the operation is regarded as a criminal act, it remains a major variable in achieved fertility (Chapter 12). In practice, abortion is available throughout the world, although where it is illegal at considerable financial, physical and emotional cost to the woman concerned.

Abortion has the most adverse political side-effects of any family planning method, but in many ways the lowest logistic costs. Experience in the Philippines shows that women may travel 3 to 5 km to obtain contraceptive services. In the case of abortion, women will travel great distances if they know their problem can be solved, and the costly promotion of services is rarely necessary. In most societies abortion services can be financially self-sufficient. With the exception of the desperately poor, most traditional farming societies and most urban poor can and will pay up to one week's disposable income to terminate a pregnancy.

The mechanical techniques for abortion in the first trimester of pregnancy are unlikely to change significantly. As with the sewing machine or bicycle, it is possible to assert with reasonable confidence that the technology has come near its final resting place.

In countries where abortion is illegal, menstrual regulation may have a particular potential. In Latin America, as pointed out in Chapter 12, abortion is only a crime if pregnancy can be proved. Even where menstrual regulation is illegal by a strict interpretation of the law, some countries are permitting responsible, open and financially accessible services to develop.

* In Korea, a saying has developed which illustrates the cultural acceptability of menstrual regulation. Equipment was imported in cartons labelled MR Kits. It is now said, 'If Dr Lee can't help you, Mr Kits will!'

All late abortions carry a higher risk, and therefore require skilled personnel and well-equipped institutions. The fact that there are a number of competing techniques suggests that no adequate technology has yet been developed. The best way of treating late abortion would seem to be to make sure the option of early abortion is readily available.

Fortunately, there is one aspect of abortion on which all groups can agree: a woman who has an illegal abortion deserves humane treatment of any complications; she has demonstrated her fertility, and is in need of contraceptive advice. Over the past decade vacuum aspiration has proved the most effective treatment of incomplete abortion (commonly the result of illegal interference), often eliminating the need for overnight stay in hospital. The post-abortal insertion of an IUD has proved safe and effective.

There is an urgent need to improve the care of women suffering from the consequences of illegal abortion. A million such women enter hospital in Latin America each year.

THE POPULARITY OF STERILIZATION

The current decade may see more sterilizations performed than at any time before and after in history. A backlog of demand from older couples must be met as well as providing for the emerging demand from younger couples. Already, sterilization is becoming the single most-used method of family planning in the world. Sterilization has proved acceptable wherever it has been made realistically available (Figure 3), but in many communities there is still political hesitancy to set a forthright policy of elective sterilization. Characteristically, the method is usually first made available to women over 30 with four children. With the passage of time this so-called '120 rule' is relaxed and women with smaller families and eventually younger age groups are 'permitted' to have the operation.

The various modalities of fertility regulation carry different economic costs in production, service and promotion. At a pure fiscal level, the choice of sterilization is probably more cost-effective than the continual supply and resupply of the reversible methods of contraception. However, it is never necessary to make a choice between these options because they should draw upon different skills and structural systems within the society, and each offers such powerful long-term economic returns to the community that it is justifiable in its own right.

Male sterilization is easier to perform than female sterilization and has been successfully carried into remote areas at relatively little cost. It seems unlikely that significant improvements or changes will be made in vasectomy.

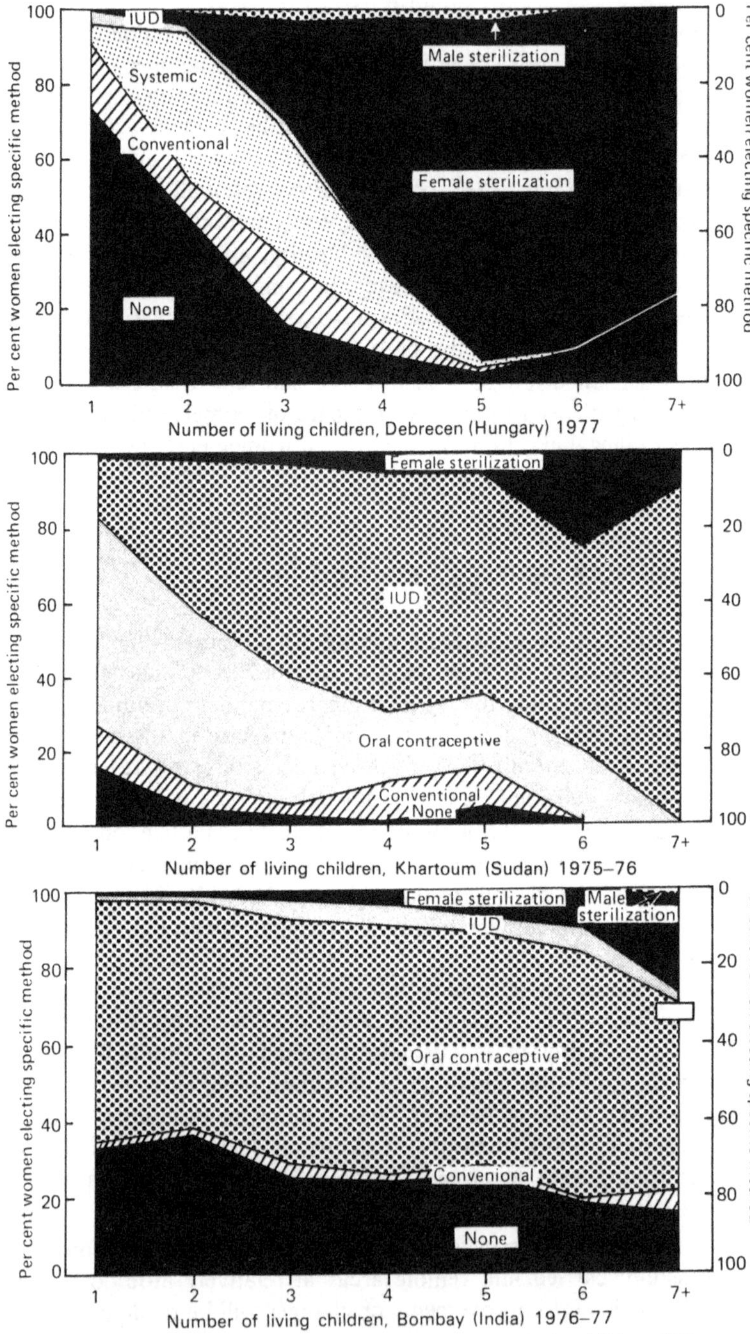

Figure 3 Postpartum contraceptive profile by method and living children

Female sterilization is a different matter. The fact that a number of competing methods are available suggests that no one is outstandingly successful. However, even at the present time and given these limitations, it has proved possible to carry sterilization services into rural areas on a discontinuous basis. Camps in India and mobile teams in the Philippines meet the need to deploy surgical expertise on a temporary basis to rural areas where it is not normally available. Kamheang has taught female sterilization by minilaparotomy through a process of decentralization from a metropolitan hospital (Ramathibodi, Bangkok) to primary, secondary and subsequent generations of satellite institutions in over 200 provincial areas, and all inside a 36-month timetable. On an average, each trainee performed five minilaparotomies, after assisting at 15. When total costs are divided by the 40 000 operations completed, the cost per case is under $US 15. When it is remembered that the average female sterilization gives 10 years or more of secure protection against pregnancy, this programme, although using a technically demanding technique in family planning, is among the most cost-effective in the world.

FUTURE AND PRESENT METHODS

No method of family planning is totally satisfactory for everyone and every method has some followers, no matter how unattractive it may appear to others. New methods of contraception would undoubtedly assist in solving family planning problems. However, the lead time on the basic research, development and testing of contraceptive methods is considerable.

Research involves looking for the unknown but this does not mean that it is a totally unpredictable field. It is possible to identify those aspects of human reproduction which are likely to be open to artificial restraint and interruption. There is no doubt at the present time that a number of biological mechanisms have not yet been translated into contraceptive techniques. Eventually, they are likely to be explored and some of them may well produce novel and acceptable contraceptive techniques. However, some may not come to fruition before a further doubling of the world's population.

There is a need to balance an appreciation that investment in basic research is the only long term strategy for improving contraceptive technology (Chapter 15), with a realization that sudden, unexpected improvements in contraceptive and sterilization technology are unlikely and the immediate need is to use the available methods as effectively as possible (Chapter 13). In the short term, policies which will permit the rational use of existing methods of family planning seem more likely to lead to better choices for individual couples than fundamental breakthroughs in technology. However, improvements in existing methods, as pointed out in Chapter 13, are advisable. Even the long-neglected vaginal barrier methods of contraception are open to improvement. Clinical trials are being conducted with spermicide-impregnated sponges (with up to 30% dry sponge weight of the spermicide nonoxynol 9) which can be left in the vagina for some time. In certain situations they could prove a useful additional method of family planning. IUDs need to be developed to meet particular situations. Encouraging results have been obtained with specially modified post-partum IUDs, which have biodegradable extensions to hold the device in place while the uterus returns to its normal size after delivery. It has been shown that if an IUD is inserted after unprotected intercourse, but before implantation has occurred, then it will prevent pregnancy. Such a post-coital method could be useful and is without the dangers that may attend the use of post-coital oestrogens.

The demand for voluntary female sterilization is so strong in many traditional societies that a concerted effort is required to develop new technologies, particularly ones that will be simple and cheap to apply (Chapter 10). Ultimately, the injection of chemicals into the cervix that will pass up and cause occlusion of the fallopian tubes would provide the optimum method – after all there are already a great many people available who can insert instruments into the cervix.

The need to be able to meet the near universal demand for something to 'bring on a late period' is a second area of surgical concern. Happily, menstrual regulation (MR) appears to be a near ideal, easy-to-teach, straightforward, safe procedure that requires no more than a clean room and a supply of simple, robust equipment costing less than $10 (Chapter 11). As is so often the case, it is policies and the law (Chapter 14) which restrain availability, not the technology itself. A pharmacological method of achieving the same end could be even more popular, especially if it could be self-administered. Even an imperfect method is likely to be widely used and could by itself bring about major policy shifts. Prohibition became impossible when anyone could make gin in his bathroom; and restrictive abortion laws would become equally redundant if prostaglandins, or other self-administered abortifacients, become readily available.

A method not dealt with earlier, but open to rapidly enlarging use, is that of injectable contraception – like MR it is controversial, but for different reasons. Despite two recommendations for approval from the relevant expert committee, the US Food and Drug Administration (FDA) has refused to extend the present approval of medroxyprogesterone acetate (Depo-Provera) the most widely used injectable, from treatment of cancer and certain other pathologies, to routine use as a contraceptive.

There are a number of women who have used Depo-Provera without interruption for over ten years and today probably a million women around the world use the drug as a contraceptive. Use-effectiveness is high, there do not appear to be any metabolic side effects and, except for causing highly irregular menstruation with frequent absence of periods, the drug appears to be a bland one. Previous fears about the return of fertility after cessation of use have been dispelled. It is perhaps fair to say that by a comparable stage and scale of use oral contraceptives had run into more problems. Although Depa-Provera is currently registered in over 60 countries, including 18 developed nations, and is purchased for programme use by UNFPA, IPPF and SIDA, the hesitancy of the US FDA undoubtedly raises questions about a dual standard for use: if it is not approved for American women, it is argued, then should it be given to women in Bangladesh?

All too often the nature of the decisions made concerning the introduction of new drugs is misunderstood. A drug regulatory authority cannot *prove* that a drug, or pharmacologically active contraceptive, is safe in advance of widespread and prolonged use. In the last analysis, the use of any new drug is an experiment on our own species. Observations in other animals and on small groups of people will only answer the question, 'On the evidence available, is it responsible to make this product or device available?' Use must always involve monitoring and there are always unknowns. In addition, nearly all pharmacologically active compounds do have side effects, which may be serious in a small number of people. Risks and benefits must always be balanced, as the history of oral contraceptives has shown. The balance, however, will differ in different countries, depending in the case of a contraceptive on such factors as the maternal mortality and the availability, or non-availability, of legal abortion. In the case of Depo-Provera the record of the drug in use is satisfactory, and if it is not to be registered in the USA it must raise the possibility that the criteria now being adopted are so strict that no profound new method of contraception will ever be adopted.

In the long term, changes in the means to control fertility can only come from basic research, and therefore the current decline in funding for research (Chapter 15) is disturbing. The investment in money and personnel for such research is likely to come from developed countries in particular. It is perhaps a hang-over from the once controversial nature of family planning, that although excess fertility relates to so many aspects of physical and social disease, it still receives so little attention. The annual budget of the US National Health Expenditure is $182 000 000 000 – greater than the combined budgets for all government activities in France and West Germany – yet the US government only spends the equivalent of three hours budget on reproductive research and contraceptive development. Reproductive research has an equally low priority in Europe and in addition the absolute level of funding is lower. The total budget of the British Medical Research Council is less than the administrative costs of the National Institute of Health in the USA.

DEMAND AND SERVICES

The theme of this volume has been that people will respond to realistic family planning services that are appropriately promoted. In some cases they are ahead of services. Global birth rates have fallen by nearly a quarter in the past decade (from an estimated 34 per 1000 in 1965 to perhaps 26 today). The annual additional increment in the world's population may have reached as high as 70 million in 1970, but today is declining for the first time since the Second World War. Ravenholt has calculated that if fertility rates had not decreased but had remained at the high level recorded in 1965, then an extra 32 million births a year would now be taking place.

The World Fertility Survey (which was mainly conducted in 1975) is documenting a consistent, strong demand by families all over the world to have fewer children (Table 1). Predictably, those with the most children are least likely to want more, but what may be surprising from a western perspective is that the less educated want fewer children than the educated, and the unskilled and agricultural labourer fewer than the professional groups. The immediate need in a great many countries is to improve the quality and coverage of family planning services. Any contraceptive method is only as good as its distribution. Successful programmes reviewed in this volume have shown that it is possible to deliver Pills, condoms and spermicides to the doorsteps of potential users through a network of personnel with a minimum of training, a simple system of supervision and no more physical equipment than a notebook and a bag to carry the contraceptives.

At the same time, it is notable that many of the successful programmes described go beyond family planning. Unfortunately, there are still polemicists who assert that family planning programmes are useless until socio-economic development takes place, just as there were people who may have overstated the family planning case a decade ago and promoted family planning as a panacea for all economic and social ills. In truth, family planning is an essential component of socio-economic change, complementary to other efforts

TABLE 1 Percentage of women who want no more children

	Country			
	Dominican Republic	*Korea*	*Pakistan*	*Thailand*
All women	45	72	49	57
Women with two children	33	66	30	46
Women with four children	62	92	69	82
Women with no education	54	88	50	66
Women with college education	28	70	46	21
Husband unskilled	46	64	—	69
—agricultural	53	75	—	61
—professional and managerial	22	72	—	43

Data from World Fertility Survey (1975–76)

to improve the economy, increase literacy, change the status of women, control disease and give dignity to human existence.

An aspect that may be new is what Mechai Viravaidya has dubbed 'fertility-related development', that is the use of contraceptive distribution as a starting point for many aspects of development. The control of human fertility is non-seasonal, affects nearly all adults and produces visible, relatively rapid change. In Thailand, Indonesia and the Philippines, parasite control has been added to family planning (Chapter 5) – an initiative supported by Japanese assistance. In Egypt, literacy and family planning have been combined. Rural credit and contraceptive distribution are to be mixed in Karnataka, India. An exciting new frontier is opening up. While community involvement and the linking of development and fertility control have been emerging themes over the past decade, an opposite trend has also become visible – involving *'disincentives'* to large families and even compulsion.

Pai (Chapter 7) has dealt straightforwardly with the role of incentives and the possible need for legislation to limit family size. As he notes, during Mrs Gandhi's 'Emergency' rule (1976–77), four states passed laws relating to compulsory sterilization when a couple had three or more children. It is also pointed out, although it is useful to state again, that not one of these bills passed into law and received the signature of the president of India. What happened during the Emergency was that in an effort to reach targets within the structure which then existed, large numbers of men in some parts of India were rounded up and vasectomized. Undoubtedly brutalities took place, and there were riots and deaths. None of these activities had the backing of law, and the tragedy is that they occurred in a situation where in other parts of the country there was still a demonstrable unmet need for sterilization, and where other options of fertility regulation, such as the Pill, were still not available to the population.

Philosophically, some people would accept compulsion over family size as preferable to the consequences of unregulated population growth. The questions that arise are: is compulsion necessary and can it be applied with justice? The first question can only be answered when every method of voluntary fertility regulation has been made available in an economically and geographically accessible way and in a culturally appropriate fashion.

This volume has underscored the fact that the fullest range of methods is rarely used, even today. None of the programmes described above involved any form of disincentive. The clinic project described in India (Chapter 7) is interesting in that people paid for a sterilization, although in other services incentives for acceptance were paid by the government. In relation to the second question – could compulsion be applied with justice across frontiers of wealth – it has to be admitted it would be difficult to implement laws compelling a restriction of fertility with the type of visible social justice necessary to make such a law acceptable in a poor country.

CHOICE

In summary, a considerable amount is known about how to make family planning services available and acceptable in a wide variety of cultures and economic settings. The major bottlenecks facing programme managers are the degree of political backing they receive in their own countries and problems with the transmission of resources.

It is recognized that many potential donors, particularly governmental and intergovernmental agencies, have to work within certain restraints. The record from the field suggests that the freedom to follow businesslike management principles, to adjust the programmes and therefore budgets to meet new demands and opportunities, and the degree of security and confidence which field personnel feel in the donor are all essentail elements to success. Attention has to be given to constructive ways of bridging the potential gap between the political and bureaucratic constraints within which many donors

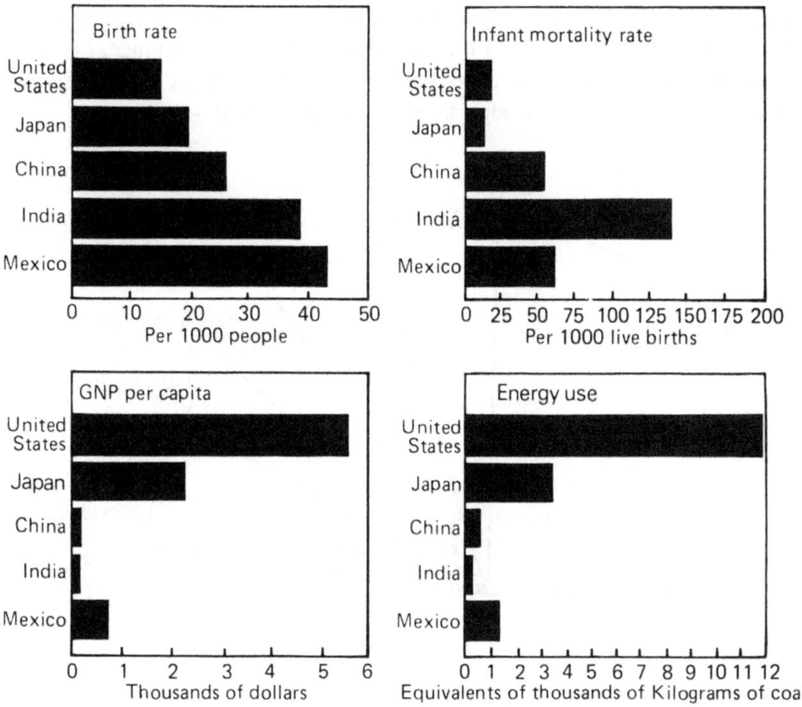

Figure 4 The development gap, 1975

have to work and the need for freedom and flexibility, which are essential to successful family planning programmes.

Although there are encouraging signs that fertility is declining in many places, hundreds of millions of couples still live beyond any type of family planning service. Differences in fertility continue to widen the gap between rich and poor; the difference between a society that can insist on schooling and create job opportunities and one where illiteracy and unemployment become chronic problems; a society where security and leisure are familiar and one where peasants toil and the exploitation of the shanty town seems inescapable (Figures 4 and 5).

Family planning extends choices to individual couples. It adds a new freedom to life. In areas where experts have predicted family planning would be controversial, it has proved to be acceptable. In places where people thought it would not be used, people have been surprised by the strength of response from within the community. All demographic considerations apart, the extension of family planning services is becoming perhaps the single most important factor in reducing maternal and infant mortality from the high levels still prevalent in many developing countries. It is a rewarding subject to work on in human terms and an exciting one because of the pace of change, the ever-expanding opportunities, and the scope for us to learn from experience and attempt to apply that knowledge to improve and adjust services.

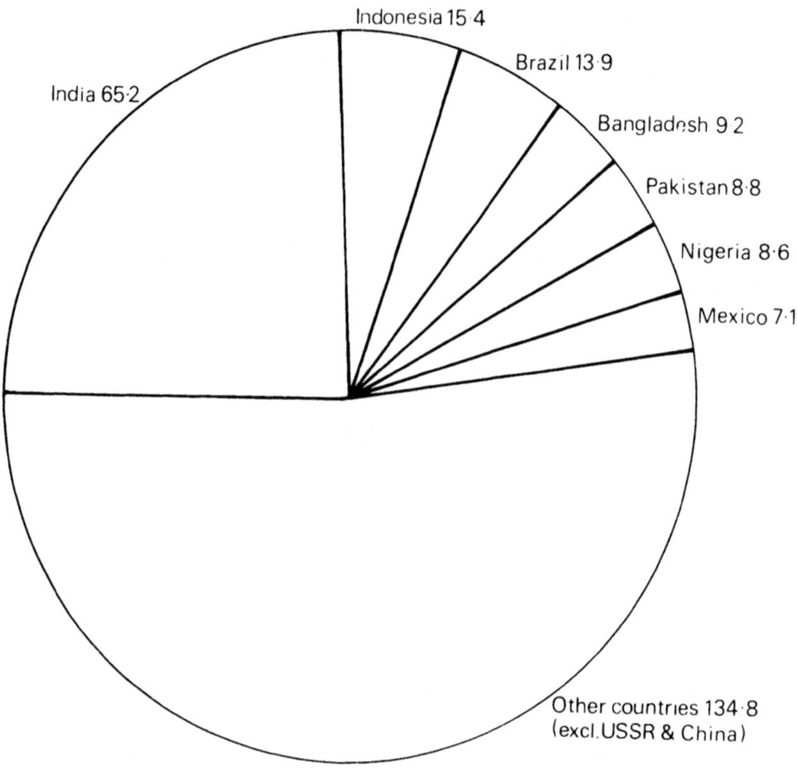

Figure 5 Women at risk of pregnancy unprotected by contraception (millions). (i.e. These are the number of women aged 15–44, multiplied by a factor of 0.628 to allow for proportions sterile or sexually inactive, and for the time necessary to achieve three desired pregnancies. Source: IPPF Survey of Unmet Needs in Family Planning, 1971–76. In: *People,* Volume 5, Number 3, 1978.

Index

Abortion
in Chile, 202, 205
complications as a result of illegal, 209
cost of to medical services, 206–7
effect of on fertility, 202–4
family planning programmes to check, 212
and fertility central techniques, 224
induced, 7
Joint Program for the Study of (JPSA), 191
in Latin America, 288, 289
and the law, 241–50
application of, 245–6
approval procedure for, 244–5
and conscientious objection clause, 245
equipment for, 248
indications for, 241–2
legal provisions for services, 242–5
legality of incomplete, 248
performance of, 242–4
protection of services, 246–7
reform of, 248
test cases, 249
legal, 210
and menstrual regulation, 188–9
morbidity and mortality in, 205–6
in the Philippines, 288, 289
solutions for eliminating, 208–11
and sterilization in Thai family planning programmes, 89
variations in pattern of, 204–7
Workshop of the Strategy for Management in Africa, 207–8
Africa
menstrual regulation in, 283
voluntary sterilization in, 237
amenorrhoea
and location, 43–5, 49
postpartum, 28, 219
Androgens, 219
Association for Voluntary Sterilization (US), 287
Austria, prosecution for voluntary sterilization in, 237
Bali, family planning programmes in, 8, 56–70
banjar system in 60–3
components of, 59–60
contraceptive services in, 59
cultural tradition in, 66
emphasis on IUDs in 60, 67, 68, 69
Family Welfare Association in, 69
history of, 57
menstrual regulation in, 63
National Family Planning Coordinating Board in, 58–9
reasons for success in, 65–9
total fertility rate (TFR) in 57, 63, 64
Bangladesh, family planning programmes in 8, 287
availability and acceptability of, 148–9
performance of programmes, 149–50
cost-effectiveness in, 149–50
self-sufficiency in, 150
promotion of, 148
social marketing barriers in, 147
sterilization in, 180, 283
Banjar system, in Bali, 60–3
frequency of *banjar* meetings, 61
Birth intervals, and lactation, 41–3
Blue Lady (Norinyl) pills, 77
Bombay, 281
incentives and disincentives in family planning programme, 125–6
overcoming fears in programme, 122–4
Pearl Centre, 127, 128
sterilization in, 121–4
camp approach, 121–2
railway station surgeries, 121
Breakthrough bleeding, 220
Breast, 220–2
Breast feeding (see lactation)
Britain, 281
and the law, 280
British Medical Research Council, 294
Bucharest World Population Conference (1974), 5, 267
Calcutta, contraceptive distribution in, 8, 102, 282
Canadian Eskimo study, 46

Center for Population Research (CPR), 257
Chile
  abortion in, 202, 205
  contraceptive distribution in, 233
  San Gregorie family planning programme, 204, 205
  surveys of women in, 203
Chronic gonadotrophin (HCG), 223
Coitus interruptus, 7, 277
Colpotomy, 182
Community-Based Distibution (CBD), in Japan, 159–62
  educational materials in, 160
Community-Based Family Planning Services (CBFPS), in Thailand, 74, 90
  fertility decline in, 83
Community Health Volunteer (CHV), 112
Condom
  distribution in Japan, 158–9
  distribution in Thailand, 85, 233
  Preethi, 139, 141, 143, 144, 145
  Raja, 148
Consumers, in Thailand family planning programme, 79–81
Contraception
  and lactation, 48–51
  and the law, 228–35
  Population Council's International Committee for Research (ICCR), 259
Contraceptive
  demand for in Japan, 159
  distribution in Calcutta, 8, 102
  distribution in Chile and Fiji, 233
  distribution in Japan, 158–9
  distribution restrictions on, 232–3
  free versus payment, 107–8
  future development of, 222–5
  injectable (Depo-Provera), 8, 89, 111, 292, 293
  male, (222–3)
  method in Howrah CBD Project, 98–100
    supply depot, 96
  methods postpartum, 50
  oral, 50, 148
  prescription requirement for, 229–32
  services in Bali family planning programme, 59
    use in, 62
  steroids, effect on lactation, 221
  use in developing countries, 4
Couple registration form, 99
Cryosurgery, 183
Culdoscopy, 182
Czechoslovakia, and voluntary sterilization, 239

Dacca, menstrual regulation in, 196
  Conference on (1975), 198
Denmark, and voluntary sterilization, 238, 239
Depo-Provera, 8, 89, 111, 292, 293
Dharma Dutta Foundation, 59, 63
Distribution restrictions,
  on contraceptives, 232–3
Dominican Republic, family size in, 4
Draper, William, 7

Eire, vasectomy in, 280
Eugynon, 77

Family planning programmes
  availability of, 271
  in Bali, 8, 56–70
    components of, 59–60
    cultural tradition in, 66
    emphasis on IUDs in, 67, 68, 69
    history of, 57
    reasons for success in, 65–9
  in Bangladesh, 8, 287
    availability and acceptability in, 148–9
    performance of programme, 149–50
    promotion of, 148
    social marketing barriers in, 147
    sterilization in, 180, 283
  and child health, 21–3
    birth interval effect, 22
    parity and birth order effect, 21
    effect on intellectual development, 23
    pregnancy timing, 22
  in China, 9, 10
  development gap in, 297
  failure of in Middle East, 32
  health rationale for, 20–1
  in India, 117–21, 295, 267
    statistics, 120
  and infertility, 29
  integration with health services in Howrah, 112
  in Japan, 154–62
    objectives of, 154–5
    budget for, 167

and maternal health, 24–6
maternal mortality, 24–5
non-obstetric conditions in high parity, 25
obstetric risks in high parity (multiparas), 25
in preventive scheme to check abortions, 212
promotion as success factor, 277–9
techniques, 278
range of methods in, 279–80
in San Gregorie (Chile), 204–5
self-sufficiency in, 282–3
services, 30
in Sri Lanka, 8, 276, 287
evaluation of programme, 142–6
implementation of programme in, 138–9
market research in, 137
performance of programme, 139–42
social marketing targets in, 138
and teenage pregnancy, 26–7
problems and hazards, 27
in Thailand, 8
background to, 72–4
administration of, 88
achievements in contraceptive use, 86
consumers in, 77–81
donor assistance, 75–6
condom distribution in, 85
demographic changes in, 82
humour in, 79–81
objectives of description of, 76–9
rural health problems in, 74
source of funds in, 87
sterilization and abortion in, 89
Family size, in developing countries, 4
Family Welfare Association (in Bali), 69
Female Sterilization, 174–84
Fertility
decline of in developing countries, 4
effect of abortion on, 202–4
future control techniques, 224
impact of child loss on level of, 31–2
immunological control of, 223
International Research Programme (IFRP), 6, 96, 199
and Mortality Survey, 66, 67
natural methods of regulation, 217
world profile of, 18–20
Fiji, contraceptive distribution in, 233
Follicle Stimulating Hormone, (FSH), 223
France
abortion in, 246
IUD insertion in, 234–5
and voluntary sterilization, 236, 237
Ford survey, 257, 261

Gonadothropin, chronic, 223
Gonadotrophin Releasing Hormone (GnRH), 224

Honolulu Conference, on menstrual regulation (1973), 63, 198
Hormone
Gonadotrophin Releasing (GnRH), 224
Luteinizing (LH), 223
Thyroid Stimulating (TSH), 223
Howrah CBD Project, 94–114, 281
background to, 95–6
barriers and bottlenecks in, 109–11
delivery system in, 96–7
community involvement in, 97–8
contraceptive method in, 98–100
economic aspects of, 106–9
evaluation of, 104–6
operation of, 100–4
depot holders in, 101, 105
depot and supplies in, 103–4
follow-up and referral in, 102
supervision, 103
shortcomings and strengths in, 113–4
Human reproduction, safeguards for, 32, 33
Human sexuality, 215–7
Hungary, IUD insertion in, 235
Hysterectomy, as a sterilization procedure, 181

Immunological control of fertility, 223
India
Council for Medical Research in (ICMR), 260
current plan in family planning, 120–1
demographic problems in, 116–7
family planning programmes in, 117–21, 295, 296
introduction of IUD, 119
legislation to limit family size in, 126–7
solutions to population control in, 129–32
strategy, 130–1

services, 132
targets for, 131–2
and voluntary sterilization laws, 239
Indonesian Planned Parenthood Association (IPPA), 57
Infertility
healthier state of, 218–22
postabortion, 206
in sub-Saharan Africa, 29
International Development Research Center of Canada (IDRC), 260
International Fertility Research Programme (IFRP), 6, 96, 199
Menstrual Regulation Study Protocol, 191
International Planned Parenthood Federation (IPPF), 5, 283, 286
International Pregnancy Advisory Services (IPAS), 12, 197
Iran, sterilization in, 180
Italy, and voluntary sterilization, 237
IUD
accepted after menstrual regulation, 198
in Bali, 60, 67, 68, 69
effects of, 50
introduction of in India, 119
legal requirements for insertion, 233–5
legalization in Japan, 162
legalization in South Korea, 234
Lippes loop, 57
postpartum, 292

Japan
CBD system in, 159–62
educational materials in, 160
demand for contraceptives in, 159
distribution of contraceptives in, 158–9
legalization of IUD in, 162
objective of family planning movement in 154–5
spousal consent in voluntary sterilization, 239
statistical information in, 163–9
budget for family planning, 167
and UNFPA, 268
Japanese Family Planning Association (JFPA), 12, 280
annual budget of, 168
current status of, 162
establishment of, 155–8
Japanese Organization for International cooperation in Family Planning (JOICFP), 162
Joint Program for the Study of Abortion (JPSA), 191

KAP (knowledge, acceptance and practice) research survey, 140, 141
'Kazoku Keikaku (Family Planning) newsletter, 156, 157–8
Kwashiorker, 20, 22

Lactation (breast feeding), 7, 217
and amenorrhoea, 43–5, 49
limitations of in extending, 44–5
and birth intervals, 41–3
menstruation and pregnancy rates, 42–3
and contraception, 48–51
decline of, 45–8
consequences for fertility, 46–7
consequences for infant mortality, 46
effect of contraceptive steroids on, 221
and health, 28
incidence and duration of, 38–41
full and partial, 40
and postpartum abstinence, 40, 41
Laparoscopy, 182
Laparotomy, 182
Latin America
abortion in, 288, 289
community-based services in, 282
Law, the
and abortion, 241–50
and contraception, 228–35
and menstrual regulation, 250–2
Lippe's loop, 57
Long-term prescriptions, technique of, 232
Luteinizing Hormone (LH), 223

Malaysia, family size in, 4
Maya, oral contraceptive, 148
Menstrual regulation, 188–200, 292
and abortion, 188–9
acceptance of, 195–8
in Dacca, 196
acceptance of IUDs after, 198
in Africa, 283
in Bali, 63
complications in, 193
cost-effectiveness of, 198–9
Dacca Conference (1975) on, 198
efficacy of, 194–5

Honolulu Conference (1973) on, 63, 198
kits, 197
and the law, 250–2
performance of, 189–95
safety in, 191–4
Study Protocol, 191
Menstruation, return of an pregnancy rates, 42–3
Methyl-2-cyanoacrylate (MCA), 183
Minilaparotomy, 181, 182, 291
Monogamy, 216
Mortality/Fertility Survey, 66, 67

National Family Planning Coordination Board (Bali), 58–9
Neosampoon spermicide, 279
Nepal, family size in, 4
Nonoxynol, 9, 292
North American Indian women study, 46, 47

Oestrogens, 219, 220
Oligospermia, 223
Oral contraceptive (the Pill), 50, 148
Ovariotexy, 183
Overseas Development Ministry (ODM), Britain, 260

Pair-bond, 216
Pakistan, family size in, 4
legalization of IUD insertion in, 234
Panama, and voluntary sterilization, 239
Pearl Centre (Bombay), 127, 128
Philippines
abortion in, 288, 289
and importance of contraception in, 281
parasite control in, 295
and voluntary sterilization, 236
Pill, the (see Oral contraceptive)
Planned Parenthood Association of Thailand (PPAT), 74, 75
Polygamy, 216
Polygyny, 216
Pomeroy method, 181
Population
future trends in, 271–2
problems, 1–3
solutions to control in India, 129–32
services, 132
strategy, 130–1
targets for, 131–2
Third inquiry, by UN, 271
total international assistance, 286
World Conference on, Bucharest (1974), 5
Population Centre for Research (CPR), 257, 267
Population Council's International Committee for Contraceptive Research (ICCR), 259
Population Services International (PSI), 8, 136, 138, 287
Postabortion infertility, 206
Postpartum amenorrhoea, 28, 219
Postpartum contraceptive methods, 50
Postpartum IUDs, 292
Preethi condoms, 139, 141, 143, 144, 145
Pregnancy rates, and return of menstruation 42–3
International Advisory Services (IPAS), 12, 197
Prescription requirements, for contraceptives, 229–32
technique of long-term prescriptions, 232
technique of signed and countersigned prescriptions, 231
technique of standing orders, 231
Progestagens, 219, 220
Progesterone, 221
Prostaglandins, 191, 251
'Proud Pete', 80, 81

Quinacrine, use of in sterilization, 183

Raja condoms, 148
Research
expenditure, 258, 259
professional personnel and facilities, 263
in US, 256, 257, 260, 262
Rhythm method, 218
Rockefeller family, aid from, 256

San Georgorio (Chile), family planning programme in, 204, 205
Sanger, Margaret, 7, 281
Sexuality human, 215–17
Silicone rubber plugs, 183
Singapore, and voluntary sterilization, 236
minimum age in, 239
waiting period in, 238

South Korea
family size in, 4
legalization of IUD insertion, 234
and voluntary sterilization, 236
Sri Lanka, 8, 276, 287
evaluation of programme, 142–6
cost-effectiveness, 143–5, 146
implementation of programme in, 138–9
market research in, 137
performance of programme in, 139–42
social marketing targets in, 138
'Standing orders' prescriptions technique, 231
Sterilization
and abortion in Thai family planning programme, 89
in Bangladesh, 180, 283
in Bombay, 121–4
camp approach, 121–2
railway station surgery, 121
colpotomy, 182
culdoscopy, 182
female, 174–84
and hysterectomy, 181
in Iran, 180
laparoscopy, 182
laparotomy, 182
minilaparotomy, 181, 182, 291
new developments in, 183
popularity of, 289–91
reversal of, 184
in Thailand, 283
use of quinacrine in, 183
vasectomy, 283, 289
in Bombay, 121
in Eire, 280
voluntary, 174, 176, 235–41
Association for (US), 287
authorization by official board, 240
benefits of, 177
bottlenecks and barriers, 179–80
camps, 179
cause of, 240–1
and criminal statutes, 235–7
in Czechoslovakia, 239
demographic impact of, 177–8
in Denmark, 238, 239
in India, 239
in Italy, 237
lack of specific provisions prohibiting 237–8
necessity for, 176–8
organizational problems in, 180–1
in Panama, 239
in the Philippines, 236
in Singapore, 236
in South Korea, 236
spousal consent in, 239
trends in laws on, 238–40
taking it to the people, 178–9
in US, 238
waiting period and minimum age for, 238
in West Germany, 239
Steroids, contraceptive, effect on lactation, 221
Stopes, Marie, 7, 281
Sub-Saharan Africa, infertility in, 29
Sweden, 280

Thailand
distribution of contraceptives in, 85, 233
family planning programmes in, 8
family size in, 4
parasite control in, 295
Planned Parenthood Association of (PPAT), 74, 75
sterilization in, 283
village distributor in, 77–8
Thyroid Stimulating Hormone (TSH) 223
Tokyo Symposium, 5, 6, 11, 12, 279, 281
Total fertility rate (TFR), in Bali, 57, 63, 64

United Nations Fund for Population Activities (UNFPA), 266, 267, 270, 286
and future planning, 268–9
United States, 281
Aid to Industrial Development (AID), 260, 283, 284, 287
National Health Expenditure, 293
and reproductive research, 256, 257
and UNFPA, 268
and voluntary sterilization, 238
Association for Voluntary Sterilization, 287
Uterus, and ovaries, 218–20

Vacuum aspiration, in menstrual regulation, 191

Vasectomy, 283, 289
in Bombay, 121
in Eire, 280
Village distributor, in Thailand, 77–8
supervision of, 78

West Germany, and voluntary sterilization, 239
Workshop on the Strategy for Abortion Management in Africa, 207–8
World Fertility Survey, 3, 38, 63, 294
World Health Organization (WHO)
Special Programme of Research
Development and Research Training into Human Reproduction, 222, 259
World Medical Society, 34
World Population Plan of Action (1974), 175, 267
Bucharest Conference (1974), 5, 267

Zilla Parishads (district organizations), 124

GPSR Compliance

The European Union's (EU) General Product Safety Regulation (GPSR) is a set of rules that requires consumer products to be safe and our obligations to ensure this.

If you have any concerns about our products, you can contact us on ProductSafety@springernature.com

In case Publisher is established outside the EU, the EU authorized representative is:

Springer Nature Customer Service Center GmbH
Europaplatz 3
69115 Heidelberg, Germany

Batch number: 10607212

Printed by Printforce, the Netherlands